HOW TO CUR

# CHRONIC PROSTATITIS

### AND GET YOUR LIFE BACK

HOW TO CURE

# CHRONIC PROSTATITIS

AND GET YOUR LIFE BACK

## MARK SWAIN

First published in 2024 by Mark Swain

© Mark Swain 2024
The moral rights of the author have been asserted

A catalogue entry for this book is available from the National Library of Australia.

ISBN: 978-1-923007-78-9

Book production and text design by Publish Central
Cover design by Pipeline Design

# CONTENTS

# INTRODUCTION
# I AGED TEN YEARS IN SIX MONTHS

Hi, I'm Mark. Thanks for reading my book.

Sometimes, I shake my head in wonder that I have written a book about Chronic Prostatitis. I'm not a doctor or medical professional. I did not even like biology much at school. My background is in financial services, so a world away from that of urologists and urology.

But I am one of the millions of poor suckers (probably just like you) who contracted Chronic Prostatitis. It's a disease that ruined my quality of life and made me age ten years in six months.

As I thought about it more and more, I decided who better to write a book about Chronic Prostatitis than a regular guy who went through the hell of trying to find why he was feeling so sick and finally discovered a way to cure it? Previously I didn't even know what Chronic Prostatitis was (until I Googled it in October 2020 – more about that later) … I had never even heard the name.

This book covers all my ultimately futile efforts visiting specialists in my home country of Australia to find a diagnosis (all of them told me there was nothing wrong with me and I was okay). It also examines the terrible symptoms I experienced, ways I was able to control my symptoms, and what I did to finally obtain a diagnosis and cure.

I walk you through the detailed daily program I undertook to get better, which took serious time, money and commitment. This may seem a bit repetitive in places, but I encourage you to read it all.

It's important for you to understand the process is a long haul and takes commitment. I also share case studies of other patients I met who are navigating their own challenges with Chronic Prostatitis and how they too are conquering the problem.

This book is for people suffering with the symptoms of Chronic Prostatitis, which commonly include:

- frequent urination
- back pain
- lethargy
- testicle pain
- headaches
- erectile dysfunction
- pelvic pain
- generally feeling unwell, with aches and a high temperature.

It will also be beneficial for family members and friends of men who are dealing with this illness.

It is intended to help people more accurately determine if they may have the symptoms of Chronic Prostatitis and explains what tests are needed to get an accurate diagnosis. The book is not intended for people looking for a magic pill or antibiotic or any type of 'quick fix' to cure Chronic Prostatitis and its devastating symptoms, because sadly there isn't one.

I hope this book helps you and allows you to also get your life back, like I did.

# PART I
# SYMPTOMS AND DIAGNOSIS

# 1

# WHAT IS CHRONIC PROSTATITIS AND WHAT CAUSES IT?

Chronic Prostatitis is inflammation (swelling) of the prostate gland. It can be very painful and distressing, with major long-term health effects.

## What is the prostate gland?

The prostate gland is a small gland between the penis and the bladder. It produces fluid that's mixed with sperm to create semen.

The word 'prostate' comes from the Greek word 'prosta', which means 'protector'. Essentially the prostate is the protector and guardian of the male sexual capacity and is a key generator of urinary efficiency and overall body energy flow.

Anything that impacts or affects the ability of the protector has a material impact on a male's energy flow and sexual confidence. This is in particular why Chronic Prostatitis is such a challenge for younger men in their twenties and thirties whose main protective organ controlling sexual capacity and activity is affected. It is debilitating for a young man who has been feeling healthy, fit and virile to suddenly feel older and lethargic. This decline in health and sexual performance is emotionally savage.

## What is Chronic Prostatitis?

The disease is essentially an infection, inflammation or disease of the prostate. Harmful bacteria or microbes have entered the urethra and found a comfortable home in the prostate. These bacteria can enter the body through sexual intercourse or contamination; for instance, by urinating in dirty sea or river water. You could even contract it by touching a surface contaminated with germs and then touching the end of your penis. I have met patients who contracted Chronic Prostatitis at their local swimming pool. Basically, anything that causes germs and bacteria to enter the male urethra can start Chronic Prostatitis.

*How Chronic Prostatitis enters and starts in the male body.*

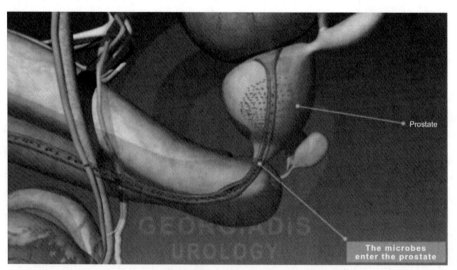

Chronic Prostatitis is the end result of a series of inflammatory reactions in the prostate gland that in turn affect the entire genito-urinary system.

Despite what many doctors and publications say, from interviewing many others who suffer from Chronic Prostatitis, I am convinced there is only one type and that is Prostatitis caused by bacteria.

That may seem like a strong statement, especially if you were told otherwise, but I explain later in the book, and also highlight the presence of bacteria in my own body and in all the patient case studies.

The bottom line is whether it's called Chronic Pelvic Pain Syndrome (CP/CPPS), Chronic Bacterial Prostatitis, Chronic Prostatitis, Acute Prostatitis or anything else, there is only one version and it is caused by bacteria.

I know this because I suffered the symptoms of all of these medical names that are bandied around. It was all eventually traced back to bacteria in my prostate causing inflammation.

Chronic Prostatitis is nearly always caused through bacteria in the urinary tract entering the prostate. The urinary tract includes the bladder, kidneys, the tubes that connect the kidneys to the bladder (ureters), and the urethra.

The inflammatory reactions of Chronic Prostatitis are caused by a variety of germs, including coliforms, enterococci, staphylococci and proteus. In addition, other microorganisms – including chlamydia, ureaplasma and mycoplasma – can cause the disease.

## Symptoms of Chronic Prostatitis

Chronic Prostatitis affects everybody in slightly different ways and every case is unique. Symptoms depend on the bacteria that has entered the prostate and its resistance level. Symptoms also depend on your age and overall physical health, diet, and a whole range of other factors. Symptoms usually start out mild and build up in intensity over time.

Common symptoms include:

- Pain, which may be severe, in or around your penis, testicles, anus, lower abdomen or lower back. Pooing can be painful.

- Sexual problems such as erectile dysfunction, sub-fertile sperm, pain during or after ejaculating, or pelvic pain after sex.

- Pain when peeing, needing to pee frequently (including at night), problems starting, 'stop–start' peeing, sometimes an urgent need to pee and sometimes blood in the urine. Also a constant urge to urinate and often a burning sensation when urinating.

- Not being able to pee, which leads to a build-up of urine in the bladder.

- Feeling as if the bladder has not fully emptied.

- Generally feeling unwell, with lethargy, aches, pains and possibly a high temperature.

- An enlarged or tender prostate.

- Headaches and migraines. Some patients complain that they are not able to work or read without an excruciating headache. Others complain of brain swelling and an inflamed head.

- Many sufferers aged twenty to thirty-five years old will show irritative symptoms such as pelvic pain, a burning sensation on urination and a sense of weight in the testicles.

- A large proportion of males aged thirty-five to fifty-five years old show more obstructive symptoms, including varying degrees of dysuria (painful urination) and often an enlarged prostate gland.

- Some sufferers also experience fever and chills.

- Occasional back pain, caused by spasms from the pelvic muscles which reflect to the back (sometimes during sleep), originally triggered by affected nerves inside the prostate.

This is what causes many practitioners to consider it a muscular issue, but with very vague explanations as to what started the pelvic spasms in the first place.

The symptoms of Chronic Prostatitis can have a significant impact on quality of life.

Recent studies have indicated 65% to 70% of the male population suffer chronic inflammation of the prostate. Prostatitis accounts for about two million visits to healthcare providers in the United States each year.[1]

Cases of Chronic Prostatitis generally depend on many factors, including the time the bacteria have been present. Key cases are usually segmented as follows:

- urgent
- moderate
- self-denial.

Let's take a look at each.

## Urgent

The sufferer experiences various intense and persistent symptoms of Chronic Prostatitis inflammation. They typically attempt to seek immediate medical treatment, often looking desperately for a radical solution because of the degree to which the condition has impacted on their quality of life.

## Moderate

The sufferer experiences moderate symptoms, annoying enough to eventually warrant a visit to a urologist. Inadequate and often incorrect assessments however lead to ineffective treatment. Persuaded that no satisfactory cure exists the sufferer accepts that somehow

---

1  Barry MJ, Collins MM. 'Benign Prostatic Hyperplasia and Prostatitis'. In: Goldman L, Schafer AI, eds. *Goldman's Cecil Medicine.* 24th ed. Philadelphia: Saunders; 2011: 805–810.

the condition is the new normal. Maybe 'it's just because I'm getting older' is a typical sufferer's response. But as their condition deteriorates, they again begin to look for solutions.

## Self-denial

This group does not recognise or does not want to pay attention to various small or moderate symptoms that begin to occur progressively. Many will undergo surgery sooner or later, either for hyper plasma (the enlargement of an organ or tissue caused by the increase in the reproduction rate of cells, often as an initial stage in the development of cancer) or prostate cancer, because the condition was not treated properly and in good time.

# 2

# CONTROLLING THE SYMPTOMS

It took me a long time to discover ways to control the symptoms of Chronic Prostatitis. I'm sharing what I have learned early with you in the book so you can at least try to reduce any pain or inflammation you have. If you are anything like me, you would do anything to subdue all the horrible symptoms you have from this disease.

## Diet

It is critical to avoid sugars, spicy foods, carbohydrates and alcohol, which any microbes in your body absolutely thrive on. They have a comfortable protected place to live in your prostate; do not make them more comfortable and give them the ability to multiply by feeding them the things they like.

If you are suffering from Chronic Prostatitis or the symptoms, you can start the following diet with immediate effect. It will not cure you, but the symptoms should subside and you will feel better than you currently do. I include them to help you here.[2]

---

2    Always seek professional medical advice before making any major changes to your diet.

# Nutritional guidelines for Chronic Prostatitis sufferers

## Fruit, liquids and juice

Drink plenty of water.

You can eat fresh fruit but avoid the very sweet ones and their juices. Specifically preferred are green apples, pineapples, kiwi fruit, mangos, plums, cranberries, berries and bilberries, pomegranate and lemon.

*Strictly avoid: Soft drinks, alcoholic beverages, packaged fruit juices that contain sugar, bananas, strawberries, cherries and dried fruit.*

## Cheese and dairy

You should prefer low-fat milk and Greek yoghurt with probiotics. Also prefer cheeses that are low in fat and salt (for example, mizithra cheese, anthotyro, cottage cheese, Milner and katiki domokou).

*Avoid: Whole milk and yoghurt, hard white or yellow cheeses, soft yellow cheeses that are high in fat. Butter and creams.*

## Vegetables

Prefer salads with fresh or boiled vegetables. You may have zucchini, carrots, broccoli, cauliflower, potatoes (roasted or boiled), spinach, lettuce, cabbage, parsley, dill, onions, leeks, artichokes, green beans, okra, tomatoes and cucumber.

Prefer virgin olive oil. Tumeric, cloves, various herbs (for example, oregano, rosemary, basil), lemon and vinegar.

## Spicy food and spices

*Strictly avoid: Hot spices and very spicy food. Avoid chili and spicy peppers. You may instead use a bit of cayenne pepper.*

*Avoid: Very salty foods, salted meat or fish, pickles and salted dry nuts.*

## Fish

Prefer to eat fish along with vegetables (for example, carrots, mushrooms, tomatoes, okra, greens, zucchini).

*Avoid: Salty and salted fish.*

### Meat and poultry

You may eat red meat, chicken and eggs.

*Avoid: Smoked meat and fish as well as canned and cured meats. Avoid low-quality seed-derived oils, fried potatoes and chips.*

*In addition, avoid packaged foods and snacks, even if they do not contain much sugar or fat.*

### Legumes and soups

You may have legumes (for example, beans, lentils, chickpeas). Prefer homemade soups with vegetables, pulses, rice, etc.

In addition, you may have unsalted dry nuts such as walnuts, almonds and cashews.

### Starch and pasta

Prefer wholegrain pasta and bread, as well as wild rice.

*Avoid: White bread, white flour, white rice, packaged pureed foods and ready-made packaged soups.*

### Desserts

You may have cake and other (unsalted) desserts made with brown flour, fruit or fruit juice, stevia and olive oil.

*Strictly avoid: Sugar and patisserie sweets. You should avoid biscuits, pastries, crackers and bakery products that contain sugar.*

*In addition, avoid chocolate milk and packaged sweets found in stores.*

## Acupuncture

Acupuncture involves the insertion of very thin needles through your skin at strategic points in your body. A key component of traditional Chinese medicine, acupuncture is most commonly used to treat pain. Increasingly, it is also being used for overall health, wellness and stress management.

I talk in detail later in this book about my journey with acupuncture. What I can say with confidence is it definitely helped me control some of the symptoms of Chronic Prostatitis.

* * *

I know not all Chronic Prostatitis sufferers have the time and money immediately available to begin a thorough prostate treatment program. Alongside your diet, consider weekly acupuncture treatment combined with daily Chinese herbs from a qualified acupuncturist to help minimise the symptoms.

# 3

## MY STORY

I was fifty-two years old as I started writing this book in Athens in October 2022. I was born in 1970. As I mentioned before, I'm a regular guy who spent many years working in financial services sales. I tell you this because I want to give you a flavour of my life before the disease.

I've always been a social and sporty guy who enjoyed life to the maximum.

My twenties growing up in the UK were a time of working hard, partying even harder and travelling the world whenever I could afford it. There were a few steady girlfriends along the way, but I was mostly out to have fun.

My thirties were spent in Australia, where I moved with my job. Life is very social down under and most events centre around having a beer. I loved moving to Australia and liked partying and chasing women even more. I was all or nothing. I'd drink vodka and Red Bulls until 5 am and stay in the next night and cook grilled fish and vegetables.

*Travelling in Borneo in my twenties (that's me at the back). On reflection, probably not the best place to urinate to avoid catching Chronic Prostatitis.*

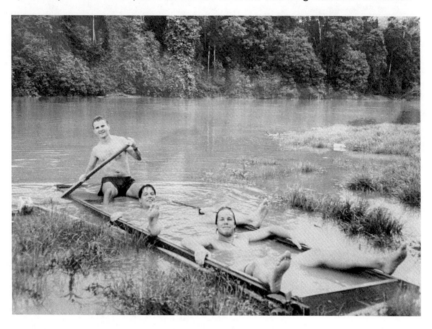

*Being in Australia was a constant rotation of work, partying and sport.*

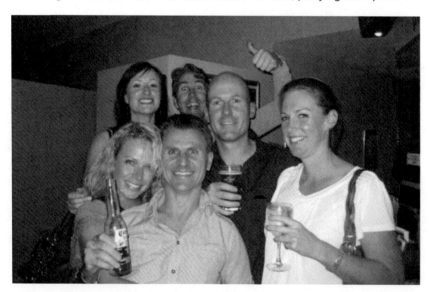

I was healthy and fit. Could run 14 km in just over sixty minutes, played tennis three times a week and was generally very sporty. I was athletic and healthy, worked hard in a relatively stressful sales job, and enjoyed weekly binge drinking to have fun and destress.

In my forties – well, at thirty-nine – I met a lovely lady Jessica who lived in Singapore. We started seeing each other regularly and are still together as I write this. I toned things down in my forties but would still have blowouts to destress from work.

In summary, over the years, I worked hard, partied hard, travelled when I could and had numerous sexual encounters, often unprotected (like most single guys do). I give you this background information to give you an idea of my prior lifestyle. I have no clue when or how I contracted Chronic Prostatitis, or more accurately the bacteria that caused it. It could have been peeing in that dirty river in the jungle or having unprotected sex with someone after a full day of drinking at the horse racing.

What I do know is at the age of forty-nine, in 2019, things started to change for me, quickly.

## The problems begin

### November 2019

Around November 2019 (nearly three years before I was diagnosed with Chronic Prostatitis), I started to notice pain in my left flank which ran down to my left testicle. This is where my expensive, frustrating and demoralising journey to finding out what was wrong with me started.

As you'd expect, I began by visiting my local general practitioner and doing a blood and urine test. I thought maybe I had a urinary infection, but the doctor said the blood and urine tests were okay and I had nothing to worry about. He gave me some antibiotics, just in case I did have a mild urinary infection.

## January to March 2020

From January to March 2020 I was not feeling myself. Often I was very lethargic, and I continued to have pain in my left flank and left testicle. In February 2020 I was visiting the Philippines to attend the wedding of my partner's best friend. I was noticing stronger left flank pain and was convinced I had a urinary infection of some kind. I purchased some strong antibiotics over the counter (as you can in the Philippines) in the hope my strong pain would go away.

After that trip, I went to the UK to bring my Mum out for a six-week holiday to Australia. This was just as the COVID-19 clouds were gathering, and we arrived the day Australia shut its borders to international visitors, 22 March 2020. I mention this because my mother has anxiety and spends lots of time worrying about things that have never happened. This causes me stress, and always has. My mother always being in a state of high alert puts me on edge too.

## April and May 2020

This stress (confirmed later by my urologist) was likely the trigger for my advanced symptomatology of Chronic Prostatitis. During April and May 2020 new symptoms started to emerge, which included my right ear blocking like I had an ear infection. My left flank pain also became noticeably stronger. I visited an ear, nose and throat specialist who examined my right ear and confirmed everything was perfectly okay. I was also starting to feel extremely lethargic and tired.

## June 2020 to August 2020

During this period my symptoms seemed to get even worse. My lower left back started to generate terrible pain. It hurt tremen-dously for me to even get out of bed.

My left flank was still bad, and I was starting to feel swelling in my head and get headaches. My head felt foggy and I just did not feel as sharp as usual. I was starting to struggle with my motivation and confidence.

Around this time, I went to see a rheumatologist to check my back and posture. I thought maybe working from home during the pandemic was starting to have an effect on my body. Again, another consultation to be told you are okay, there is nothing wrong with you!

Are you starting to see a common theme here? *You are okay.*

## September and October 2020

By this time I was starting to feel noticeably older. It was as if I had aged ten years in six months. I started thinking to myself, *well I am fifty years old now, maybe it's just the ageing process.*

In October 2020 I was referred to a top Sydney urologist by my doctor. During my consultation I had my first 'finger up the bum' experience. The urologist inserted his gloved finger into my backside and began pressing and feeling my prostate. His conclusion; there is nothing wrong with it. According to him my prostate was a good size and texture. I paid my $250 for a thirty-minute consultation and left his practice even more confused and anxious about what was wrong.

It was around this time that I tried to exercise my way through the lethargy. I would hit the gym three or four times a week for a strong cardio, stretching and overall weights body workout. The weird thing was my back was aching and painful when I went in for the workout and hurt just as much or more when I walked out. I just knew something was wrong.

The lethargy at this point started to get ridiculous. I would wake up after ten hours of sleep absolutely exhausted, with a fuzzy head. Often surfacing around 7 am and having a morning swim and breakfast, sometimes I had to go back to bed at 10.30 am absolutely exhausted. Now is that normal? Is that okay?

It was around this time I was visiting my local doctor again, who this time sent me off for scans on my abdominal area, testicles and kidney. Everything was all clear (a relief) apart from a very minute kidney stone that I was advised would not be causing any pain or issues.

By October 2020, my back pain was becoming excruciating. I struggled to get up in the morning and could not even bend down to pick up a golf ball. I was also noticing my head swelling even more and liquid started to come out of my ears. I would get this weird sensation like an insect was wriggling around in my ears.

My fatigue was terrible by now and I said to my partner Jessica:

'I cannot keep living like this – I'm really struggling.'

I felt miserable, old and very low.

It was around this time I started to Google my symptoms (as you do). Fibromyalgia, Chronic Fatigue Syndrome and Chronic Prostatitis were three possible options that came up. I was also concerned, given my level of fatigue, that I had picked up an infectious disease such as Dengue Fever or some weird river-related insect disease you read about. I booked an appointment to visit the infectious diseases ward of Sydney Royal North Shore Hospital and explained to the specialist doctor about my lethargy, inflammation in the head, wriggling in my ears and back pain. I did more blood tests and had a long discussion, but my results were all clear according to the specialist. She said it is probably just stress related to COVID-19 (which by October 2020 was starting to spread around the world). Her opinion was it is a very anxious time for everybody, but don't worry – you are okay.

When you get told so many times you are okay and you know you are not, you start to question yourself and put all of your declining health down to getting older.

It was at this point – and with Sydney now starting to have lockdowns and restrictions – that I emailed Dr Pavlos Georgiadis in Athens, who I found on Google as a Chronic Prostatitis Specialist. Below is the first email I sent to him.

Hi Pavlos,

I trust this email finds you well.

I noticed some of your work on the internet and wanted to reach out.

Over the last 6-9 months I have been getting pain in my left testicle and lower left back.

The pain started this January in my left flank area and then progressed to my left testicle and lower left back.

Sometimes the pain in my lower back is excruciating and I've taken Nurofen (which seems to help) these last 3 weeks.

I have had my spine scanned, blood and urine tested with no problems and a check for a hernia.

I know I'm based in Australia but am starting to struggle given I'm normally extremely fit. I'm 50 years old, non-smoker and 74 kg athletic/slim build.

Please reach out if you feel you can help or if you have ideas you can help me with.

I'm in Sydney and happy to have a virtual consultation given Covid.

Regards

Mark

Below is the reply from Dr Pavlos Georgiadis in Athens on 13 October 2020. As you can see, he was able to diagnose my likely Chronic Prostatitis over email.

Dear Mr Swain,

First of all, thank you for your message and good evening from Athens. With regards to what you mention:

The testicular + lower back pain are indicative of Chronic Prostatitis (CP) too.

The intensity of the pain is very common as well.

Given that you have confirmed the lack of other factors, it is very likely that it is Chronic Prostatitis.

If you want to confirm it, you would need to perform a Transrectal Ultrasound from a specialized Urologist with radiological training + semen & sperm culture microbiological exams (but again, the doctor needs to know how to press the prostate before, and you would need to know how to condition yourself). Unfortunately, there is widespread ignorance about CP around the world, so even if you get negative results, do not automatically assume that it is the case.

In all honesty, I would recommend you come to Athens when the times are convenient and safer, and I examine you myself + potentially begin CP treatment (assuming that's the case, which is very likely). Until then, the most substantial thing you can do is **careful diet and lifestyle**. Avoid sugars, spicy foods, alcohol and in general anything that would increase inflammations. Unfortunately, I cannot do much more remotely, but if you have any questions, please do not hesitate to ask and I will try to answer them when I can.

Kind regards,

Dr Pavlos Georgiadis

And here is my response on 13 October. At this stage I was in Australia and unable to travel internationally.

Thanks so much Pavlos for your response.

If indeed I do have CP would it be OK adopting a healthy lifestyle until I'm in a position to get to Athens?

In other words, is it OK if I leave it 6-9 months and focus on a healthy diet and plenty of water?

Kindest regards

Mark

Here is the doctor's email response on 19 October 2020 advising I should adopt a healthy lifestyle to try to contain any likely Chronic Prostatitis.

Dear Mr Swain,

Good evening from Athens. With regards to your questions:

A healthy lifestyle will definitely help with keeping inflammations low, but the inflammation as well as the microbes will still be there. However, there are some things to keep in mind:

Several transformations still develop inside the prostate, even if delayed.

This can be either additional symptoms or sudden worsening of current symptoms.

If additional complications exist, which may not be apparent now (e.g. urethral strictures, pelvic pain spikes, hyperplasia, diminished quality of erections, etc.), it is a matter of time for them to get aggravated and become more established, leading to more necessary work.

The existing microbes create the conditions so that further microbes can establish themselves in the prostate, and survive against the body's natural mechanisms.

In any case, from my side I can treat any CP at any stage that I receive it, but naturally the longer the patient has had the condition (and the more the complications), the more time it takes to restore the prostate tissue as well as the possible complications.

In full honesty, I would recommend that you visit me as soon as you can and it is safe to do so, and indeed until then try to follow a healthy lifestyle strictly.

I hope this helps.

Kind regards,

Dr Pavlos Georgiadis

By October 2020 I was probably at my lowest point and was experiencing a multitude of symptoms, which in order of the worst first were the following:

- Excruciating lower right back pain, making it difficult to get out of bed. It hurt to pick a golf ball out of the hole and normal movements were constantly painful. The pain would also be on my lower left side sometimes as well. My partner constantly worried about me groaning like an old man getting out of bed.
- Left flank pain. Sometimes sharp but usually a dull, constant pain.
- Horrible lethargy and fatigue. Little motivation to do anything physically or mentally strenuous. However much I slept I never felt refreshed.
- My right ear kept blocking like I was on an airplane at 36,000 feet. It felt like I had an ear infection.
- I had left testicle pain that kept coming and going: a sharp type of pain sometimes and dull at others.
- My head felt like it had inflamed and swelled up. I sometimes had a feeling of my heart beating in my head loudly when I laid down or after a hot bath.
- Numbness in my right thigh – I didn't feel anything when I touched it lightly.
- Stiffness in my neck and back.
- Pins and needles in my feet sometimes when I woke up.
- Thick yellow coating constantly on my tongue.

These were my symptoms, but all cases are unique and many other symptoms of Chronic Prostatitis are often present.

## 2021: A year of acupuncture and Chinese herbs to reduce the pain

By the end of 2020 my back pain was excruciating, my ears were regularly blocking, my head was swelling up, liquid was starting to run out of my ears sometimes when I was asleep and my left flank pain was worse.

## I was a lethargic, tired mess.

An athletic, fit, dynamic, positive guy, full of energy had become a negative old man who had aged fifteen years in one year.

One day I was playing tennis against some sixty- to seventy-year-old guys who were still pretty fit, and I was the one who had to come off the court because my back had locked up, my muscles were tight and it hurt to move around the court. The pain was just too much.

What was going on with me? Why was I needing to leave a tennis court playing guys twenty years older than me? I remember thinking if ageing happens this fast, then by jeez it's bad! I thought, *this situation is getting desperate, what can I do to get my old life back?*

While playing this game of tennis and having to leave the court in excruciating pain, I remembered how the local Chinese acupuncturist had cured my tennis elbow some eight to ten years ago. I left the court and called the acupuncturist straight away. I was in luck – there was a space for an immediate visit.

Chinese acupuncture dates back thousands of years and is an ancient practice where needles are inserted in strategic positions on the body to fight various illnesses and diseases, including chronic fatigue, digestive problems, menstruation problems, infections, migraines, anxiety and depression.

In January 2021 during my initial meeting with Doris Chen from the Harmony Clinic in Manly, Sydney, I had a detailed consultation. Doris listened to me intently describe my symptoms in detail. I explained my lifestyle, what I had been through in the last year, and how my life had become miserable.

*How Chinese acupuncture is used to target inflammation and disease in the body.*

# HOW ACUPUNCTURE WORKS

## SIGNAL STIMULUS

The stimulus from acupuncture needling creates a cascade of signaling throughout the connective tissue (fascia) involving the blood, nerves and immune system.

## ACUPUNCTURE NEEDLE INSERTION

- Stimulates a local and a centralized reaction.

- The local reaction involves Sensory Neurons in the skin being stimulated.

- The central reaction occurs when the signals reach the brain and spinal cord.

## ACUPUNCTURE POINTS

Acupuncture points are located in areas with higher concentrations of:
- Superficial nerves
- Blood vessels
- Neuromuscular attachments – where vessels and nerves penetrate muscle fascia

## CENTRAL EFFECT OF NEEDLING

Both the Central and Peripheral Nervous Systems are effected

NERVOUS SYSTEM

| Central Nervous System | Peripheral Nervous System |
|---|---|
| Brain | Voluntary Muscles – movement |
| Spinal Cord | Nerves |
| HPA Axis (see below) | Smooth Muscle – lining of organs |
| | Stress/Emergency response |

## WHAT YOU REALLY NEED TO KNOW

1. Acupuncture needling promotes homeostasis and self-healing. In short, acupuncture stimulates the body to heal itself.

2. Acupuncture influences:
   A. The Nervous System — muscles, nerves, internal organs

   B. Cardiovascular System — blood flow, distribution of nutrients, hormones

   C. Endocrine System — Hypothamlic-Pituitary-Adrenal axis regulation– major pathway for homeostatic regulation

   D. Immune System — strengthens the immune function of the body

I'd never had any doctor or specialist up to this point listen to me with as much concentration as Doris did. After thirty minutes of just listening to me explain my host of symptoms and problems, including my ski trip to Japan in 2020 where our accommodation was absolutely freezing, she had a diagnosis:

## I had a blocked liver meridian and fluid trapped on my lungs.

Doris said she could help me get rid of my back pain, and the pain in my left flank and left testicle. She was the first specialist who said to me 'you are not okay' and she was able to help me.

I started my first acupuncture program immediately, on 7 January 2021. Doris placed needles strategically in my left flank, abdomen and legs. What I found freaky about this first treatment was the needles when inserted swiftly brought out the exact symptoms of a bad cold I'd had when skiing in Japan some nine months earlier. When I was lying down on the massage couch getting more needles in my back (near my lungs) and legs, my nose just started to stream out liquid and I came straight out with the same bad cold I'd had while skiing.

After my first acupuncture, Doris gave me some Chinese herbs to take daily with hot water.

My acupuncture program carried on every Monday for sixteen months up until May 2022 (when I was able to leave Australia and take my Mum back to the UK). I would drink my daily herbs – for which the ingredients were carefully selected each week according to my progress – either once or twice a day after meals.

*The liver meridian is an ancient energy channel in the body, according to Chinese acupuncture. It controls energy flow, digestion and more.*

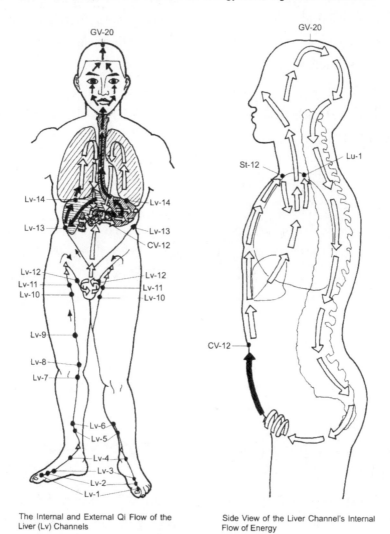

The Internal and External Qi Flow of the Liver (Lv) Channels

Side View of the Liver Channel's Internal Flow of Energy

Acupuncture helped me, but it didn't cure me. I'm sure it reduced the inflammation in my body, and I know it largely eliminated my lower back pain. I'm confident it helped me have a year somewhat less miserable than 2020.

However, despite all my disciplined acupuncture treatment, daily herb intake and stopping drinking alcohol, I was still experiencing:

- extreme lethargy
- swelling in the brain/head
- intermittent left flank pain, sometimes sharp
- feeling old and not dynamic
- ears blocking and wriggling sensation in my ears
- thickish yellow tongue coating
- beating sound in my head quite regularly, especially when my head first hit the pillow at night.

As I moved into 2022 (and with Australia now opening its borders fully) I was looking forward to my first holiday after nearly two-and-a-half years of lockdown. My last acupuncture was on 19 May 2022, before boarding a plane to take my mother back to the UK on 22 May 2022.

How would I feel without the weekly acupuncture program?

I wasn't really looking forward to the flight given I already had swelling in my head and blocked ears. The trip however was okay and it was nice to be back at my Mum's house in the village where I grew up – Silverstone in Northamptonshire, UK.

I still wasn't 100% myself when I was in the UK and I didn't have the same physical ability to play golf like I used to when visiting. I used my time in the UK to do some jobs around my Mum's house, but quickly got tired doing simple tasks like clearing out the garage and gardening.

During a weekend with a friend in London in late June going to Wimbledon and to watch Duran Duran in Hyde Park, I felt pretty tired and sluggish the whole weekend (I'm sure the alcohol was not helping). I came back to Northamptonshire on Sunday evening on the late train. Upon waking on Monday, I felt wretched.

My body was aching terribly and I could not get out of bed. I'd contracted COVID-19 while in London. For some reason COVID-19 hit me particularly hard, much worse than friends who contracted it. It turns out that the Chronic Prostatitis in my body was already causing my immune system to be very low and inflammation was already present. COVID-19 just took things to a whole new level, and it was six weeks before I could walk for an hour. I thought I was pretty healthy, but obviously at this stage I was not.

I'd largely recovered from COVID-19 by late August, although I still felt pretty weak and jaded. I was, however, certainly looking forward to a holiday in Greece, after two-and-a-half years in Australian work-from-home isolation and the same amount of time living in an apartment with my anxious mother and girlfriend.

# 4

## BEING DIAGNOSED WITH CHRONIC PROSTATITIS (FINALLY)

I arrived in Athens on 1 September 2022 to meet up with an old UK work friend from American Express in Brighton.

Arriving on Thursday night, we were straight out to eat some pizza and hit an Irish bar to drink some long overdue catch-up pints. Over the next few days, we hit the best bars and clubs Athens could offer. It was a pretty constant stream of pub grub (think steak and ale pies and Cajun chicken burgers) and mojito cocktails and more Guinness. On reflection, probably the worst possible diet for a Chronic Prostatitis sufferer!

I have always generally thought my lifestyle was pretty healthy. I never eat fast food, don't drink canned sugary drinks, don't smoke, and don't eat lots of sweet desserts. I do however like traditional English food, including English breakfasts, spicy curries, fish and chips and occasional apple crumbles. I would also regularly eat vegetables, chicken and fish, and always had boiled eggs or high-fibre bran for breakfast.

*Me departing London for Athens for a well-deserved vacation.*
*I thought I looked pretty healthy and well. Little did I know!*

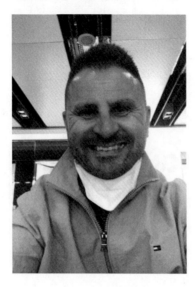

After three nights in Athens seeing the sights and visiting more restaurants and bars, the pain in my left flank was getting worse. At one point after more Guinness and pub food at the James Joyce Irish Bar in Athens, I had a really sharp pain in my left flank going right into my rib cage.

In advance of my trip, I had taken a chance and randomly emailed the doctor I had communicated with back in 2020:

Hi Pavlos,

I hope this message finds you well.

I am actually going to be in Athens for 6 days from this Thursday evening.

I am still getting lower back and left flank pain.

Should I come and see you for a consultation while I am there? Please let me know what is involved with the initial consultation.

I will be then back in Athens after 3 weeks following a visit to some Greek Islands.

Please let me know when you are available and I will come say hello.

Regards

Mark

And the doctor's reply:

Good morning Mr Swain,

You could come on Monday morning at 11.30 to start with the exams (ultrasound transrectal, Flowometry and microbiological tests).

So avoid urinating after 9 am on Monday and take care to avoid ejaculation at least 3 days prior to the appointment.

Let me know if everything is ok with you to fix the appointment.

Have a nice day.

Pavlos

## The initial consultation

I felt I had nothing to lose by visiting the doctor while I was in Athens. I also had a pretty free day on that Monday, before we were due to go to the Greek Islands of Serifos and Milos for five days.

Upon arriving for my appointment at Dr Georgiadis's surgery, I was struck by how professional everything was. The clinic was modern, clean and professional.

The doctor had asked me in advance to attend the appointment with a full bladder so I could perform a flow test of my urine. I was waiting in the reception having a water-drinking competition with fellow new patient Stratos to see who would be the first to visit the doctor and have his urine flow measured.

When I did meet Pavlos for the first time it was evident he was an expert in the field of Chronic Prostatitis. I explained all my long-standing problems to him, and he explained it was probably the restricted prostate causing a trapped nerve that was causing me all the back pain. However, he would need to do a full transrectal scan of my prostate, scan my kidneys, bladder and urethra, and measure my urine flow to determine if Chronic Prostatitis was actually the cause of my problems.

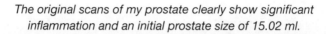

*The original scans of my prostate clearly show significant inflammation and an initial prostate size of 15.02 ml.*

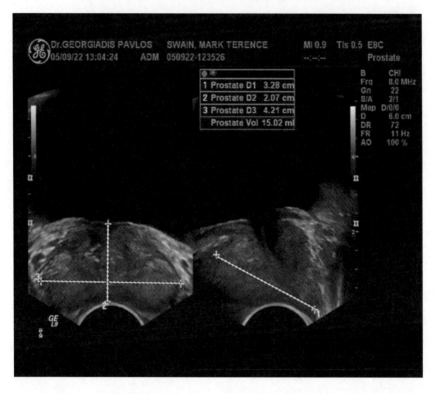

Below is the original uroflow test of my urination measurements. It shows a disrupted, volatile flow of urine. This was being caused by inflammation in my prostate and urethra and the likely presence of bacterial microbes. I joked with the doctor that this urine flow looked like a very volatile stock market chart!

*The original test of my urine flow shows*
*a disrupted, volatile flow.*

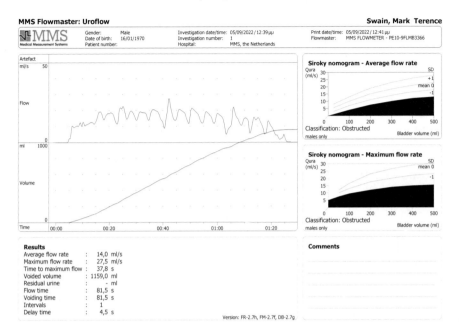

After showing me the scans included here, Pavlos advised I needed to start treatment immediately if I wanted to improve my health and prostate and get my life back. He said I had left things too long during the COVID-19 lockdowns and I really needed to start work on getting better immediately.

I'd spent many months and thousands of dollars seeing numerous Australian specialists who all told me I was okay. And here was someone who definitively tells me what is wrong and what is causing all my symptoms. He even gives me the images to prove it.

## The doctor explained I had probably had Chronic Prostatitis for over ten years.

I actually felt relief knowing I had Chronic Prostatitis because I had known all the way along something was wrong with me. We all know our own bodies, don't we?

Pavlos explained I would need to stay in Athens for daily treatment for the next six weeks to resolve my problem. I said to him I am fully committed to this – I am 'all in'.

I immediately contacted my friend to arrange to catch up for lunch and advise the boat trip to the Greek Islands was off for me. I had to get urgent treatment on my prostate. I knew deep down if I did not fully start and commit to the program now I would never do it.

\* \* \*

In the section that follows I detail week by week the treatment I went through to cure my Chronic Prostatitis. Every case is unique and different and may well be a variation on what I went through. I however am passionate about sharing my very personal and private story with you so you too can see you can cure Chronic Prostatitis and get your life back.

# PART II
# TREATMENT

# 5

## MY TREATMENT PLAN

The doctor explained I would need to undertake twice-daily treatment sessions in his surgery, once in the morning and once in the late afternoon or early evening.

### WEEK 1: Breaking down the inflammation and sclerotic tissue.

#### Monday 5 September

After my initial consultation which showed my body had an inflamed prostate and obstructed urination, the next step on day one of the program was to start breaking down the inflammation and find out what bacteria was actually causing the infection.

I was back in the surgery at 5 pm for my first prostate massage. Not knowing fully what to expect, I was asked to take down my pants and trousers and kneel on a leather stool with my core resting on a massage-style table.

*The scene of my first prostate massage in Greece. The goal was to break down sclerotic tissue in my prostate and release any microbes living there that could be analysed in a later sperm sample.*

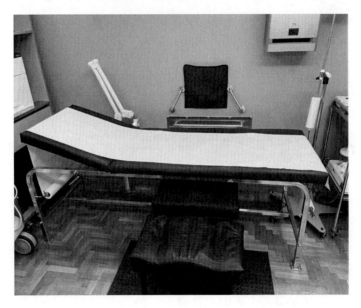

The doctor proceeded to put on one of his rubber gloves, what I later found out were colloquially called 'happy hands' gloves! He applied some kind of gel and inserted his right index finger into my backside.

He started pressing on my prostate, and it didn't feel good. He seemed to be breaking down this hard, calcified tissue inside of me. The pain was horrible, and I sweated the most I have ever sweated in my life. My T-shirt and the leather kneeling pad and table were soaked. My stomach felt nauseous and I was a bit dizzy. All the energy seemed to drain from my body. I could not believe the pain – this was just the first forty seconds. The doctor then stopped the massage for a minute, and then proceeded to do another for forty seconds more. I was hanging onto the leather cushion for dear life! That was the second forty-second prostate massage and I sweated even more.

We took another one-minute break and then the dreaded doctor walked up behind me again for massage three. Another forty seconds enduring the pain, sweating and feeling lightheaded. I had another break for one minute and then my fourth prostate massage; the doctor continued to rub and press hard all over my prostate to break down areas that had obviously hardened over time. I slumped over the table after he took his finger out of me. I was exhausted and hardly able to move. I'd completed my first session of prostate massage and it was *not* pleasant. I've never to this day experienced a pain like this, which at the same time was also a weird kind of relief for me.

After the massage and taking some time in the clinic reception to get my breath again, calm down and drink some water, I was advised I needed to do a sperm test.

I had to get a taxi to the Mycolab microbiological test centre on the outskirts of Central Athens. The clinic knew I was due for an appointment, and on arrival I paid my €210 and was given a small plastic bottle in which to deposit a sperm sample. I was shown to a room a bit like a dental clinic, equipped with a dentist's reclining chair, and was told to please put my sample in the plastic bottle. *Great! Just whip up a sperm sample like that in a Greek dentist-style laboratory*, I thought. It was hardly the most romantic setting.

Luckily, I had some battery left on my phone and the clinic had a wi-fi connection. I was able to pull up an erotic video to stimulate me. I found a movie that worked for me and managed to whip up my sample. I think if I'd had a flat mobile phone battery going into that sterile clinic I would still be there now!

The lady on reception at Mycolab advised me I would have the results from the sperm test in seven to eight days. They would be sent directly to the doctor and to me. I then took a taxi from the clinic to a pharmacy near my hotel to get the initial oral tablets prescribed for me.

I came out with a whole bag of tablets, including:

- Arcoxia, which I had to take once a day after lunch for the inflammation.
- Norocin, which I had to take first thing in the morning one hour before breakfast and in the evening one hour before my evening meal.
- Bactrimel that was taken after lunch.
- Ultra Levure and Lacto Levure probiotics that were designed to protect my stomach from the wave of antibiotics that would be coming my way.

After the sperm sample escapade and stocking up on antibiotics, it was back to the cafe next to my hotel to grab a meal in compliance with my new dietary regime.

*The first meal in accordance with my new dietary program, in the afternoon of 5 September 2022. I was so exhausted all I could muster the energy up to order was a salad and vegetables. The white bread served with it was definitely not allowed to be eaten.*

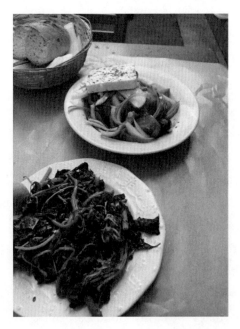

I went to the hotel exhausted from the day's demands after a brief chat with my friend. I laid on my bed that night with a mixture of emotions swirling through my head. Relief that I had my Chronic Prostatitis diagnosed and someone had finally told me what was wrong with me. Exhaustion from what had been a tough and demanding day. And some trepidation about what lay ahead. It's a date I definitely won't forget. Monday 5 September 2022. The first day of getting my life back.

## Tuesday 6 September

On day two of my program the goal of breaking down the sclerotic tissue in my prostate continued. At 10 am and 5 pm the doctor would see me for a session to massage my prostate.

I joked with the doctor that I was visiting the Theatre of Pain for my twice-daily prostate massages. His perspective was I was visiting the Athens complete body rejuvenation centre where I would become healthier and younger.

Nothing can prepare you for these first few prostate massages, which are undoubtedly the toughest. The release of toxins and bacteria and the breakdown of sclerotic tissue causes your body's central endocrine system to go into overdrive, essentially having to filter out all the harmful toxins that have built up over the years.

The prostate massages were very tough again and a real struggle to even get through. The 10 am treatment sucked all the energy out of me. I would count down each second, praying for it to finish. When I did get my one-minute break I dreaded hearing the doctor walking up behind me ready to insert his finger again. All up the prostate massage session only lasts about ten minutes, but due to how busy the doctor is it may take up to one-and-a-half hours including waiting time. One of the bonuses of waiting to see the doctor is you start chatting to other patients in a similar predicament to yourself and start forming relationships.

You rapidly learn there are so many people suffering from Chronic Prostatitis. Millions, if not tens of millions.

All I felt like doing after having my morning massage was getting a healthy lunch, grabbing a siesta and mentally recharging for the 5 pm second treatment of the day.

At 5 pm I went through the 'finger up the bum' four by one-minute treatment prostate massage again. Alongside the prostate massages I had to be very diligent about exactly when I took my prescribed antibiotics to give my body the best chance to fight the infection inside me.

Having two prostate massages a day is demanding and depleting. I'd however committed to the program to get the fastest and best treatment so I had to learn to just stick this out.

It was evident to me this early in the program that I needed to have three core capabilities to see this program through, which were:

- time
- money
- commitment.

I also quickly learned that to progress efficiently in the program and have the maximum chance of a swift recovery I needed to be:

- relaxed
- comfortable
- focused.

*How the prostate massage breaks down the hard and sclerotic tissue and starts to transition the prostate from an unhealthy, hard, stoney type to a healthier soft and spongy type.*

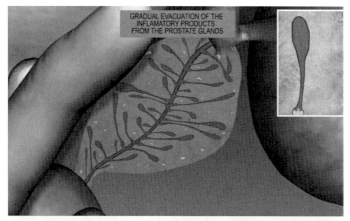

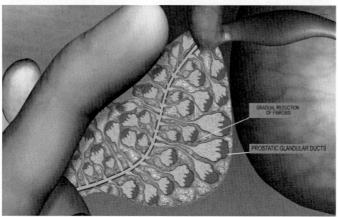

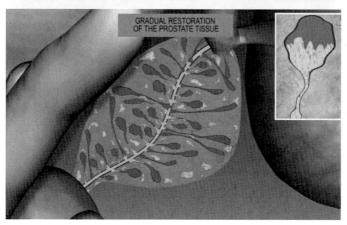

I decided to book into a comfortable mid-range hotel, the Dunlin Hotel, for the Monday to Friday nights I would be staying in Athens. I immediately came off social media to cut down on any unnecessary stress and avoid distractions during my treatment. I also vowed to be extra disciplined in complying with the dietary requirements of the program.

## Wednesday 7 September

To speed up the rejuvenation of my prostate and assist in breaking down the hard tissue, the doctor introduced daily Piezo shockwave treatment to my prostate from day three. This was in addition to my twice-daily prostate massages.

The PiezoWave machine sends an electronic pulse up through your anus to the prostate area to assist in faster regeneration of elastic muscle. It is a similar principle to treatment many of us have had to speed up recovery of a calf injury from a physio.

*Daily Piezo shockwave treatment was performed on my prostate from day three to speed up the breaking down of the hard sclerotic tissue that had built up over the prior ten years.*

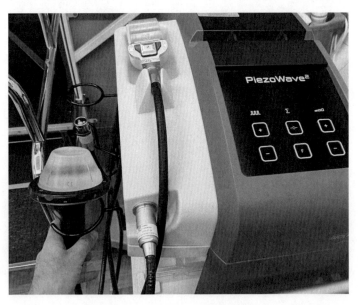

The electronic shockwave treatment was not painful. All I had to do was lay down on the massage bed on my side with my trousers down and lift my legs up, while the doctor applied gel to a rounded electro gun ready to fire into my anal area towards my prostate for ten minutes.

I continued with the twice-daily treatment on the Thursday and Friday.

I was jubilant to finish my first week of treatment on the Saturday. I cannot overstate how demanding both physically and mentally the sessions are. I had the weekend off to meet up with a friend and relax at the beautiful Astir Beach near Voula.

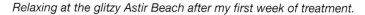

*Relaxing at the glitzy Astir Beach after my first week of treatment.*

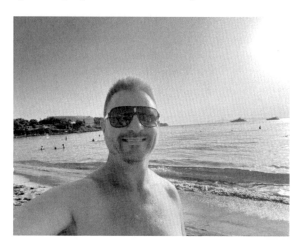

One recommendation I would make to anyone embarking on this program is this:

Book yourself something at the weekend to look forward to. It helps you mentally and physically get through each day of the program.

## WEEK 2: Finding bacterial microbes causing infection and optimising antibiotic treatment.

### Monday 12 September

My weekend relaxation came to an abrupt end with my 10 am appointment to visit the doctor, who by now I was referring to as the Terminator – he was the Terminator of microbes. This would be the week I received the diagnosis from my sperm culture examination submitted the week before.

One thing is for sure – there is nothing that has *ever* woken me up more on a Monday morning than a prostate massage. It brings a very sharp conclusion to the weekend!

I was sticking rigidly to my new diet and taking all my prescribed medications.

At the start of the second week of the program the doctor noticed I had some kind of sexual dysfunction. This was total news to me, as I'd not struggled to get an erection – but I had noticed my sex drive had diminished over the last few years, particularly during the COVID-19 period. I just thought it was because I was getting older and put it down to having less privacy with my mother staying in our Sydney apartment with myself and my partner Jessica. One of the big problems of Chronic Prostatitis is your body adapts around the deterioration it causes. As a result of the inflammation, infection and the multitude of symptoms, the body seeks to coexist with the problems and adapt to them.

The outcome is a body and mind that accepts you are deteriorating and just getting older.

Anyway, to correct the new sexual dysfunction that I'd just learned about, the doctor planned to introduce an additional treatment to my twice-daily prostate massages and twice-daily prostate PiezoWave treatment. He was going to introduce his sexual dysfunction program!

Not something a guy really wants to hear.

What happened next shocked me – literally. On the Monday evening the doctor asked me to lay down on my back on his treatment table. With my trousers around my ankles, he proceeded to put a – I don't even know how to describe it – small, gentle slice or cut into the base of my penis near my stomach.

This allowed him to fit some kind of clip to me. He then covered my penis in a lubricating gel. I could not will myself to open my eyes and look down and see what he was doing. He then proceeded to put this vibrating tube on my penis which pulsed and started to give me an erection. He used this vibration machine until I was hard.

### After this, he proceeded to carry out PiezoWave shock treatment on my penis. This was not the Greek vacation I had planned!

The penis PiezoWave sent electronic pulses through my penis that went straight up to my brain. This procedure is designed to stimulate sclerotic tissue that had built up in my penile shaft due to Chronic Prostatitis.

The results were truly stunning as the erection shockwaves made me think about every girlfriend I'd ever had, right from my first school girlfriend at fourteen years old. Go figure. All I could think about was ex-girlfriends and my previous sexual activity.

I also noticed a strong pulsing in my right ear, which I found weird as this was the ear that had been causing me so many problems with blockages and caused me to visit an ear specialist some two years earlier at the height of my symptoms.

I was on this erection electrification machine for what must have been fifteen minutes before the doctor proceeded to detach his machinery, unclip me from the device at the base of my penis and wipe the gel off me. I was ready to go back to the outside world.

When I walked out of the surgery after this sexual dysfunction treatment, I was like a sexual caged tiger. I was like a virulent, randy sixteen year old walking down the road. I just could not stop looking at any half-attractive woman on the street (and trust me, there are plenty in Athens). I was just zooming in on any nice female pair of legs, nice butt, cleavage or attractive face I could see.

I was actually struggling to comprehend what was happening to me as I walked down the road still with a semi-hard erection. Importantly, I was starting to realise the link between my prostate and other parts of my body. I would never have believed how intricately the prostate is linked to the brain and ears.

### The doctor was right: I did have some kind of sexual dysfunction and he had started to unblock it.

I continued having this sexual dysfunction treatment every day for the rest of the week, including Saturday mornings. I also was having my twice-daily prostate massages and daily prostate PiezoWave shock treatment.

### Tuesday 13 September

On the Tuesday of my second week of treatment my first sperm results came back. The sample I had submitted the Monday before came back showing I had staphylococcus aureus and klebsiella pneumoniae in my prostate. My white blood cell count of leukocytes was also very high at 35–40 per field, indicating my body was working hard fighting the infection.

*The results of my microbiological exam showing the presence of staphylococcus aureus and klebsiella pneumoniae in my sperm.*

Ιδιωτικό Διαγνωστικό Εργαστήριο Ειδικών Λοιμώξεων - Μυκητιάσεων & Μικροβιολογικών Εξετάσεων
• Τμήμα Βιοπαθολογίας (Ορμονολογικό-Βιοχημικό-Αιματολογικό-Ανοσολογικό) - Μοριακής Βιολογίας - Προγεννητικού Ελέγχου
• Τμήμα Κυτταρολογίας - Εργαστήριο Ψηφιακής Ανάλυσης Εικόνας
(Digital Image Analysis Lab)

*myc*

Λεωφ. Κηφισίας 354 Χολάνδρι Τ.Κ. 15233
ΑΦΜ:998012799 - ΔΟΥ: ΧΑΛΑΝΔΡΙΟΥ
Τηλ. 210-8028817, 210-6890505 Φαξ: 210-6890506
www.mycolab.gr - info@mycolab.gr

Patient name: MARK SWAIN    DATE: 05/09/2022

## CULTURE OF SPERM

Leukocytes (White Blood Cells):  Enough (35-40)per field
Stem Fungus:  NEGATIVE (-)
Neisser:  NEGATIVE (-)
Gramm stain:  POSITIVE (+)

**Cultivation (aerobic)**

Klebsiella pneumoniae + Staphylococcus aureus

**Cultivation (anaerobic)**

NEGATIVE (-)

**Chamydiaceae:**

NEGATIVE (-)

**Mycoplasma Fermentans**

NEGATIVE (-)

**Mycoplasma Hominis:**

NEGATIVE (-)

**Ureaplasma Urealyticum:**

NEGATIVE (-)

**COMMENTS**

Ph 8.0 - Hb (+) Erythrocytes (Few 10-12) per field

The Doctor

51

Ιδιωτικό Διαγνωστικό Εργαστήριο Ειδικών Λοιμώξεων - Μυκητιάσεων & Μικροβιολογικών Εξετάσεων
• Τμήμα Βιοπαθολογίας (Ορμονολογικό-Βιοχημικό-Αιματολογικό-Ανοσολογικό) - Μοριακής Βιολογίας - Προγεννητικού Ελέγχου
• Τμήμα Κυτταρολογίας - Εργαστήριο Ψηφιακής Ανάλυσης Εικόνας
(Digital Image Analysis Lab)

myc

Λεωφ. Κηφισίας 354 Χαλάνδρι Τ.Κ. 15233
ΑΦΜ:998012799 - ΔΟΥ: ΧΑΛΑΝΔΡΙΟΥ
Τηλ. 210-8028817, 210-6890505 Φαξ: 210-6890506
www.mycolab.gr - info@mycolab.gr

EURO
CERT

CERTIFIED MS.
ISO 9001:2015

# ANTIBIOGRAM

**MARK SWAIN**                                **Athens**      05/09/2022

Material :          *CULTURE  OF  SPERM*

Microbe :          *Staphylococcus   aureus = 80.000  cfu/ml*

| | Classif/tion | MIC's | | Classif/tion | MIC's |
|---|---|---|---|---|---|
| PENICILLINE : | | | ERYTHROMYCIN: | R | |
| AMPICILLIN: | R | | CLARITHROMYCIN: | R | |
| AMOXICILLIN: | R | | ROXITHROMYCIN: | R | |
| AMOX.+AC.CLAVUL.: | S | | AZITHROMYCIN: | R | |
| AMPICIL.+SULBACT: | | | | | |
| PIPERACILLIN: | | | | | |
| PIPERACILLIN/TAZOBACTAM: | | | AZTREOENAM: | | |
| TICARCILLIN: | | | IMIPENEM: | | |
| TICARCILLIN+AC.CLAV.: | | | MEROPENEM: | | |
| | | | GENTAMICIN: | S | |
| | | | TOBRAMYCIN: | | |
| CEFADROXIL: | | | NETILMYCIN: | | |
| CEPHALOTHIN: | S | | AMICACIN: | S | |
| CEPHAZOLIN: | | | TETRACYCLIN: | R | |
| CEFAMANDOLE: | | | DOXYCYCLIN: | R | |
| CEFOXITINE: | S | | CLINDAMYCIN: | S | |
| CEFUROXIME SODIUM: | R | | METRONIDAZOLE: | | |
| CEFUROXIME AXETIL: | R | | CHLORAMPHENICOL: | S | |
| CEFACLOR: | | | TRIMETH. SULFA: | S | |
| CEFPROZIL: | | | NITROFURANTOIN: | S | |
| CEFIXIME: | R | | ACID  FUSIDIC: | S | |

1 of 2

Ιδιωτικό Διαγνωστικό Εργαστήριο Ειδικών Λοιμώξεων - Μυκητιάσεων & Μικροβιολογικών Εξετάσεων
• Τμήμα Βιοπαθολογίας (Ορμονολογικό-Βιοχημικό-Αιματολογικό-Ανοσολογικό) - Μοριακής Βιολογίας - Προγεννητικού Ελέγχου
• Τμήμα Κυτταρολογίας - Εργαστήριο Ψηφιακής Ανάλυσης Εικόνας
(Digital Image Analysis Lab)

Λεωφ. Κηφισίας 354 Χαλάνδρι Τ.Κ. 15233
ΑΦΜ:998012799 - ΔΟΥ: ΧΑΛΑΝΔΡΙΟΥ
Τηλ. 210-8028817, 210-6890505 Φαξ: 210-6890506
www.mycolab.gr - info@mycolab.gr

EURO
CERT
CERTIFIED MS
ISO 9001:2015

# ANTIBIOGRAM

**MARK SWAIN**                    **Athens**        05/09/2022

Material :       *CULTURE OF SPERM*

Microbe :        *Klebsiella pneumoniae = 100.000 cfu/ml*

|  | Classif/tion | MIC's |  | Classif/tion | MIC's |
|---|---|---|---|---|---|
| PENICILLINE : |  |  | ERYTHROMYCIN: |  |  |
| AMPICILLIN: | R |  | CLARITHROMYCIN: |  |  |
| AMOXICILLIN: | R |  | ROXITHROMYCIN: | R |  |
| AMOX.+AC.CLAVUL.: | R |  | AZITHROMYCIN: | R |  |
| AMPICIL.+SULBACT: |  |  |  |  |  |
| PIPERACILLIN: | S |  |  |  |  |
| PIPERACILLIN/TAZOBACTAM: | S |  | AZTREOENAM: | S |  |
| TICARCILLIN: | R |  | IMIPENEM: | S |  |
| TICARCILLIN+AC.CLAV.: | S |  | MEROPENEM: | S |  |
|  |  |  | GENTAMICIN: | S |  |
|  |  |  | TOBRAMYCIN: |  |  |
| CEFADROXIL: |  |  | NETILMYCIN: |  |  |
| CEPHALOTHIN: | R |  | AMICACIN: | S |  |
| CEPHAZOLIN: |  |  | TETRACYCLIN: | S |  |
| CEFAMANDOLE: |  |  | DOXYCYCLIN: | S |  |
| CEFOXITINE: | S |  | CLINDAMYCIN: |  |  |
| CEFUROXIME SODIUM: | S |  | METRONIDAZOLE: |  |  |
| CEFUROXIME AXETIL: | S |  | CHLORAMPHENICOL: |  |  |
| CEFACLOR: | S |  | TRIMETH. SULFA: | S |  |
| CEFPROZIL: |  |  | NITROFURANTOIN: | R |  |
| CEFIXIME: | S |  | ACID FUSIDIC: | R |  |

1 of 2

I did not know what to really think when I received these results. My primary reaction seemed to be relief that I was getting to the heart of what was causing my problems and satisfaction that I was uncovering so much valuable information and progressing more positively than I had in the last two-and-a-half years.

I was also starting to feel more virile throughout week two, with erections waking me up at night and a general feeling of better health.

*By the end of week two of the program I was starting to lose weight and look noticeably healthier. My skin looked better, my eyes were sparkling and my brain felt sharper.*

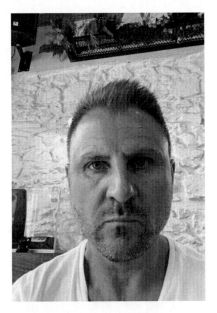

I noted in my journal at this stage the key ways I was feeling different after just ten days of treatment. The main differences I was seeing were:

- I was losing weight
- my brain had stopped swelling

- I had less left flank pain
- I had more energy
- I felt more positive
- I had firmer erections
- my ears blocked less
- my heart didn't feel like it was beating in my head
- my neck was not stiff
- I felt cleaner and fresher
- I had more confidence
- I felt and looked younger
- My body looked more toned.

## WEEK 3: First injection in the prostate to accelerate bacteria elimination.

The third week of the program would be a week where I would have my first injection in the prostate. This injection is designed to target the worst areas of inflammation in the prostate and diminish any sclerotic hard tissue there. The goal is also to promote generation of good tissues and blood vessels to start healing in areas where this can freely happen.

### Monday 19 September

On the first day of week three, the doctor did another transrectal ultrasound and uroflow test on me. It had been exactly two weeks since I started the program.

It was important to do the tests before I had the full week of intravenous antibiotics and prostate injection to allow further monitoring and analysis post-surgery.

*My second transrectal scan of the prostate showed a noticeable reduction in inflammation over the first two weeks of treatment. My prostate had also reduced in volume from 15.02 ml to 12.38 ml.*

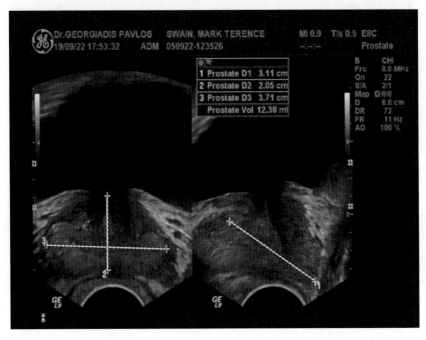

*The second uroflow test showed a reduction in the volatility of my urination.*

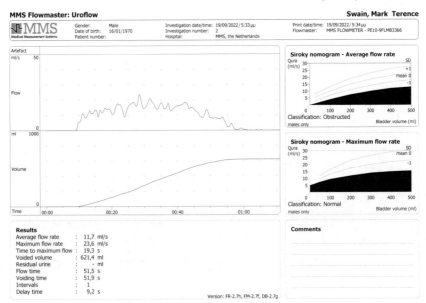

The week of the intraprostatic injection is a big, demanding week. On Monday morning I had to be at The Central Clinic of Athens at 7.30 to start my first cocktail of antibiotics that would be fed via a drip into my arm. Over a period of three hours, six concoctions of between around 200 ml and 400 ml dripped into me. Firstly, two bottles of fluids to protect my stomach, followed by the antibiotics, which on my first morning were 250 ml of Voncon, 100 ml of Meronem, 300 ml of Zyvoxid, Losec and 4 ml of Zofran. It should be noted that prior to entering the clinic I had to show a negative COVID PCR test, which in my case was taken on the Saturday morning before treatment.

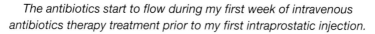

*The antibiotics start to flow during my first week of intravenous antibiotics therapy treatment prior to my first intraprostatic injection.*

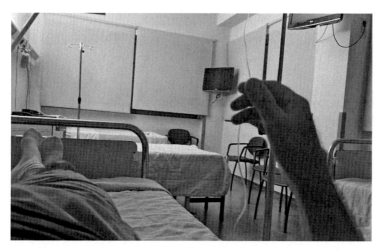

After three hours of antibiotics was a five-minute walk to the doctor's clinic where I would have my regular 10.30 am triple treatment combination of:

- prostate massage (one minute × four)
- prostate PiezoWave (ten minutes)
- sexual dysfunction erection PiezoWave treatment (fifteen minutes).

After some time for food and a light siesta I was back for the second session of the day at 6 pm, which consisted of:

- prostate massage (one minute × four)
- prostate PiezoWave (ten minutes).

At 6.30 pm I was back at The Central Clinic of Athens hooked up to more antibiotics, which slowly and steadily dropped into me over the next three-and-a-half hours. I was pretty tired by the time I got home but happy I had the needle out of my arm.

## Tuesday 20 September

The second day of injection week involved the same twice-daily trip to the doctor and the same twice-daily visit to the clinic for drip antibiotics over a total of six-and-a-half hours.

## Wednesday 21 September

This would be the big day: surgery day.

I could not eat any food for breakfast and could only have two glasses of water before heading to The Central Clinic of Athens.

Again, this involved my regular cocktail of antibiotics from 8 am to 11 am. It seemed by this stage the nurses were finding it harder and harder each day to find a vein through which they could inject the antibiotics.

I had noticed my fellow patient Tariq kept his cannula (small flexible plastic tube inserted into a vein for delivery of antibiotics directly into the bloodstream) in at night to sleep. At this stage I preferred having my needle taken out so I could move more freely and sleep better at night.

After the morning's intravenous (IV) treatment I went straight to the doctor's clinic for my regular program of:

- prostate massage (one minute × four)
- prostate PiezoWave (ten minutes)
- sexual dysfunction erection PiezoWave treatment (fifteen minutes).

After that morning's treatment I only had thirty minutes to relax in the doctor's comfortable waiting lounge before I had to be back at The Central Clinic of Athens to prepare for surgery.

*I spent many hours in the doctor's comfortable waiting room, including a well-needed thirty minutes relaxation before heading to The Central Clinic of Athens for my first prostate injection.*

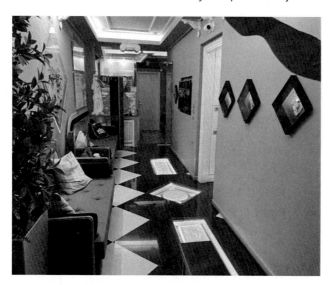

Back at the hospital clinic to prepare for surgery I had to take off all my clothes and put on an open-back hospital operating gown, hospital underwear and blue plastic socks. I could not look in the mirror as I felt I looked ridiculous without even seeing myself!

It was then all systems go. A friendly nurse came into the IV treatment room, asked me to get on his hospital wheelie bed and proceeded to push me down the aisle to the surgery area. It was when I was pushed into an elevator and transported down to the surgery floor, I thought, *shit, this is a serious program I'm on now.*

I had some blood taken out of my pelvic vein, had a plastic hairnet applied and was covered in a blanket before I was wheeled into the operating theatre.

It was a bit daunting being in a full-scale hospital operating theatre (I'd never been in one before), surrounded by probably six or seven doctors and nurses in their hairnets, face masks and green hospital operating outfits. I was relieved to see the friendly face of Doctor Pavlos who would be doing the operation and directing proceedings. The full menu of treatment I was about to have was:

- PRP prostate injection – to regenerate and rejuvenate healthy tissue in my prostate affected by long-standing inflammation.

- PRP penis injection – to regenerate and rejuvenate healthy tissue in my penis affected by long-standing inflammation.

- Intraprostatic injection – an injection of a cocktail of antibiotics into my prostate to help kill the staphylococcus aureus and klebsiella pneumonia bacteria present.

- Fibrinolytic agent – an injection of a special agent to help disintegrate hard tissue that had built up in my penis and prostate.

Before I knew it a doctor said I would start to feel drowsy soon and proceeded to inject some fluid into my arm. Anaesthetic was being injected, I felt dozy and sleepy, and was soon stone cold out in another world.

While I was relaxed in this 'other world', the world of Chronic Prostatitis correction, I had all the injections and procedures above done. The next thing I knew I woke up in the operating theatre waiting room, feeling dazed and listening to another patient next to me who seemed to really enjoy the anaesthetic ride.

After a short time to start to come around, probably fifteen minutes, I was wheeled back up to the IV treatment therapy room to rest and recuperate.

The first thing I noticed after the treatment was a pain in my backside, which was caused by a bandage that had been placed on my rear during the operation to soak up any blood and fluids. I was supposed to wait one hour before I removed the bandage, but as I was in discomfort, I went to the bathroom to take it out. When I removed the bandage lots of bloody, gooey brown liquid came out of me. At least the pain had gone, and I was able to shower there and clean myself up.

> I didn't feel any major pain after the surgery and was able to rest and recuperate in my hospital bed alongside fellow intraprostatic injection patients Tariq and Thomas.

After resting from surgery, it was back to the doctor's clinic for a prostate PiezoWave session of ten minutes. Luckily for me there would be no prostate massage that afternoon after the surgery as the doctor advised me it was sensitive and could not have any pressure applied for two or three days. I was so pleased to hear this, as I never looked forward to a prostate massage!

At 7 pm I was back at the hospital for four more hours of antibiotics and stomach support fluids, including 250 ml of Voncon, 100 ml of Meronem, 300 ml of Zyvoxid and 4 ml of Zofran. The antibiotics seemed to drip into my body slower and slower. I left the hospital clinic at 11.10 and was back in my hotel room at 11.30 pm, exhausted from my treatment that had started at 7.30 in the morning.

*Back in my room with my cannula still in after my first intraprostatic injection.*

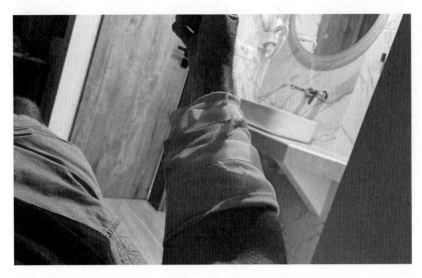

The rest of the week (Thursday, Friday and Saturday morning) were spent having my twice-daily, three to three-and-a-half hours of intravenous antibiotics and regular treatment of PiezoWaves on the prostate and penis, excluding the prostate massage.

On the Friday I also had a third uroflow test. It was performed to measure my urine flow and determine what effect the IV antibiotics and injection had on my inflammation.

I don't think I have ever looked forward to a weekend as much as this weekend, and following my final IV antibiotics and treatment on the Saturday morning I was a free man. My cannula was disconnected, and I could go and enjoy myself.

I took a boat to the idyllic Agistri Island with the sole purpose of resting and relaxing after my demanding week.

Taking time out to relax from the program on weekends for me was very important. I don't think I could have continued with as much treatment as quickly as I did if I didn't do this.

*My third uroflow test showed an improvement from before the IV antibiotics and intraprostatic injection. This demonstrated that the antibiotics were successfully targeting microbes inside my prostate and reducing any restriction in the urethra from inflammation.*

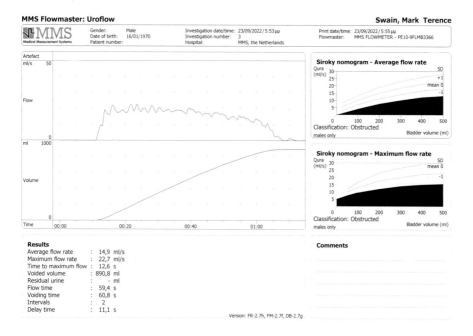

*Relaxing at the beautiful Agistri Island after my very demanding first week of IV antibiotics and first intraprostatic injection.*

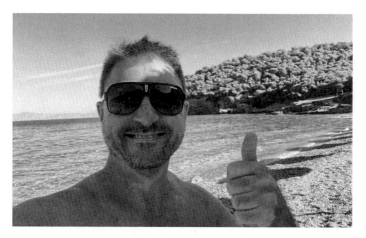

## WEEK 4: Continued breakdown of prostate inflammation.

### Monday 26 September

After last week's demanding full week of intravenous antibiotics, it was back to my regular schedule this week. The focus of treatment this week was to further break down the inflammation and hard tissue in my prostate as well as continue treating my sexual dysfunction.

> I never liked the term 'sexual dysfunction', but it is what it is.

After my lovely relaxing weekend away, I soon came back to reality. I was back in Central Athens at the now familiar Asklipiou 39 for my 10.30 am appointment with the Terminator (of microbes).

The now familiar sound of Pavlos putting on his 'happy hands' rubber gloves and applying gel while I kneeled on his leather chair bent over brought my weekend relaxation to an abrupt halt. It was time for the prostate massages to start again after my prostate injection last week. This would be my first prostate massage since last Wednesday morning, some five days ago.

While receiving the prostate massage my prostate felt sensitive (not painful) and the doctor was gentler than normal while pressing any hardened areas. The four one-minute massages on my prostate were over relatively easily.

As usual this was followed by ten minutes of PiezoWave electrification pulse treatment, placed on my anus to send shockwaves up towards the prostate. This procedure is designed to speed up the breaking down of any fibrotic tissue that has built up.

My penile erection electrification session followed, with probably ten minutes to prepare everything and ten minutes of actual shockwave treatment on my erection. I was now starting to notice a big difference in my libido and was noticing the following:

- regular erections during the night while sleeping, and in the morning
- I was feeling more virile and younger
- my sexual drive had noticeably increased.

By this stage of the program every day was starting to feel a little bit like I was doing a work project and was a bit rinse and repeat. My usual daily routine was:

10.30 am: Treatment one (prostate massage, prostate PiezoWave, penis erection PiezoWave)

11.30 am: Morning coffee at Cultivos Cafe

12.30 pm: Nutritious lunch at Nikitas

2.00 pm – 4.00 pm: Daily siesta (I found this helped me recover my energy from the morning treatment and prepare myself for the afternoon session)

5.30 pm: Treatment two (prostate massage and prostate PiezoWave)

7.00 pm: Light meal

8.00 pm: Relax in my room before bed

10.00 pm: Bed (good sleep is critical during this program)

By now I was in the fourth week of the program and noticed that the weight was dropping off me. I also looked so much healthier and younger.

I would FaceTime my girlfriend in Australia and she would say, 'You look younger every day and I look older. I want your treatment program.'

*A visual comparison of how I looked before the program and when I started week four. I was looking noticeably younger and healthier and had lost 3 kg already.*

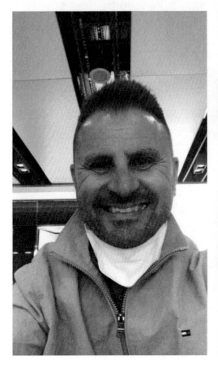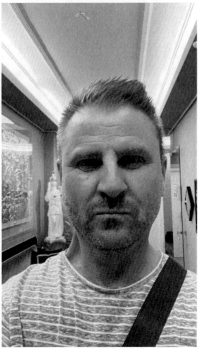

The remainder of week four was spent doing my regular twice-daily program of:

## Morning

- Prostate massage (one minute × four)
- Prostate PiezoWave (ten minutes)
- Sexual dysfunction penis erection PiezoWave treatment (fifteen minutes)

## Evening

- Prostate massage (one minute × four)
- Prostate PiezoWave (ten minutes)

After my Saturday morning treatment I was free to relax for the weekend. I picked up a hire car and headed off to the ancient ruins and coastal area of Sounio.

## WEEK 5: Start treating urinary stricture caused by Chronic Prostatitis. Continued treatment of prostate inflammation.

### Monday 3 October

One of the big problems of Chronic Prostatitis is the additional complications it can cause, especially if left over time. Longstanding inflammation starts to spread out of the prostate into the penile shaft. This inflammation affects sexual performance and the ability to urinate properly.

Early in week five of my program I was talking to the doctor and explained that the last quarter of my penile shaft felt restricted. It turns out this inflammation was the cause of me needing to urinate very frequently and often quite urgently. Again, this is the nasty work of the microbes, staphylococcus aureus and klebsiella pneumoniae in my case.

This urinary restriction was also confirmed by the fact that high doses of intravenous antibiotics improved my urine flow. When I was taking IV antibiotics the microbes were subdued or even killed, thus causing less inflammation in my penile shaft and less obstructed urine flow.

The doctor advised on the Monday morning he was going to do the first dilation to widen my urethra. Now I'm no doctor, but I didn't like the sound of that!

While I was lying on the doctor's treatment table with my trousers around my ankles, he proceeded to apply some kind of antiseptic spray into the end of my penis.

I could not even look at what he was doing, and I started to sweat and wince as he said he was going to insert something into my penis.

The doctor made some kind of very small cut down my old fellow. I can see your eyes watering now! It was designed to open the penile shaft and aid better urinary flow, and surprisingly was not painful. Or so I thought.

After the procedure I went to the toilet and literally sprayed pee everywhere – I simply could not control it. It was like I had placed my thumb over the end of a garden hose and the flow was squirting everywhere.

Worst of all, it felt like I was peeing fire. I had to grit my teeth. After spending five minutes cleaning up the doctor's bathroom I went back to see him and told him about my sprinkler session. His response was, 'Bravo – that's just what we wanted'. *I'm not sure it is what I wanted*, I thought, but I trusted him on this.

By the end of the week, I was in a position to do my fourth urine flow test to see what difference the opening of my urethra had made. The results follow. My original flow had high disruption with all the ups and downs.

My fourth uroflow test showed a marked improvement, with smoother flow, less volatility, and was starting to resemble the bell curve smooth shape it should be.

*A comparison of my first urinary flow on 5 September (top) before*
*I started the program and on 7 October (bottom) in week five.*

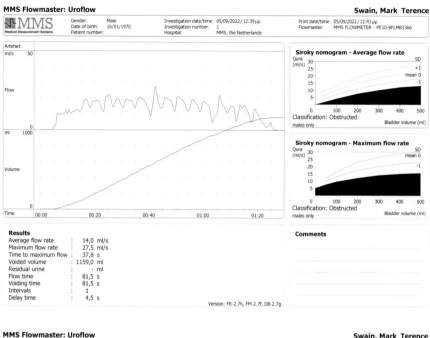

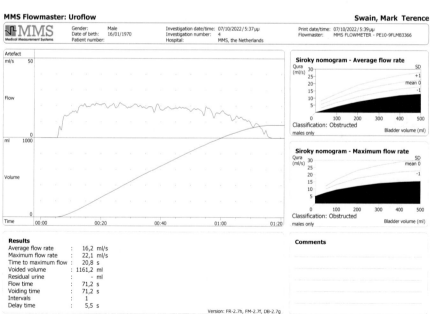

At the end of week five I also had my third transrectal scan done with new imaging of my prostate. This would show how the inflammation was reducing and how the program was working so far.

*Five weeks into the program I had noticeably less inflammation in my prostate. Due to this reduced inflammation and infection my prostate size had reduced from 15.02 ml to 11.99 ml.*

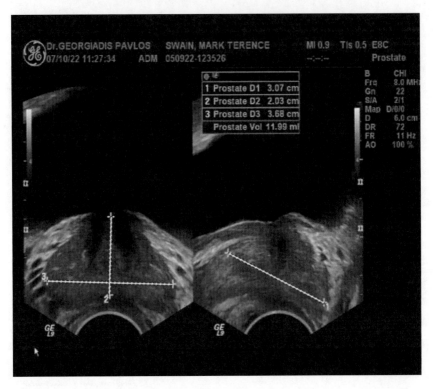

On the Saturday morning after my fifth week of treatment concluded I was straight to Piraeus Port in Athens by taxi to catch a fast ferry to the beautiful and relaxing Agistri Island again. Arriving on beautiful Agistri Island was just what I needed after my fifth week of treatment – particularly given next week would be my second intraprostatic injection and another full week of intravenous antibiotics.

*Arriving on beautiful Agistri Island*

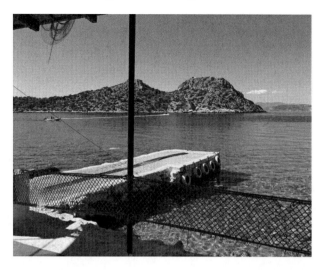

## WEEK 6: Second injection in the prostate to further reduce bacterial infection and inflammation. Urethra dilation to further increase urine flow and reduce urinary strictures.

### Monday 10 October

This would be the week of my second injection in the prostate. The injection was scheduled for Thursday, which meant I did not need to start taking intravenous antibiotics until Tuesday. Yay!

The week of the injection and constant clinic visits to do hours of intravenous antibiotics is the most gruelling part of the program. I had my normal Monday treatment program with the doctor.

### Morning
- Prostate massage (one minute × four)
- Prostate PiezoWave (ten minutes)
- Sexual dysfunction penis erection PiezoWave treatment (fifteen minutes).

71

### Evening

- Prostate massage (One minute × four)
- Prostate PiezoWave (ten minutes)

## Tuesday 11 October

On the Tuesday morning as I walked past Omonia Square in Athens to start my 7.30 am antibiotics there was the most beautiful sunrise.

*Walking past Omonia Square to start my second week of intravenous antibiotics. I would go on to joke with the Doctor that my future urine flow would be as strong as the fountains gushing water.*

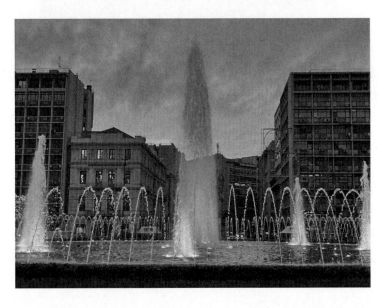

I was in the therapy ward for IV intravenous antibiotics by 7.30 on the Tuesday morning. One of the positives of the second week of IV treatment was at least you are familiar with what is involved.

I ground my way through three hours of IV antibiotics in the morning and three-and-a-half hours in the evening. My daily antibiotic cocktail was:

## Morning

- Two bottles of stomach protector
- Voncon 250 ml
- Meronem 100 ml
- Zyvoxid 300 ml
- Losec
- Zofran 4 ml

## Evening

- Two bottles of stomach protector
- Voncon 250 ml
- Meronem 100 ml
- Zyvoxid 300 ml
- Zofran 4 ml

In addition to the daily IV antibiotics, I had my regular daily treatment previously shown.

## The nurses on the ward were really friendly and did everything they could to look after me.

This week I also had my urinary flow very carefully monitored before and after the surgery. With a urethral dilation planned this week to improve urine flow it was important to measure my flow before and after surgery.

During IV week you have time to grab some lunch and a rest between 1 pm and 4 pm before returning for the second treatment of the day and second intravenous session.

*During week six of the program my second week of intravenous antibiotics started. Every day was an early start at 7.30 am and a late finish around 10.30 pm.*

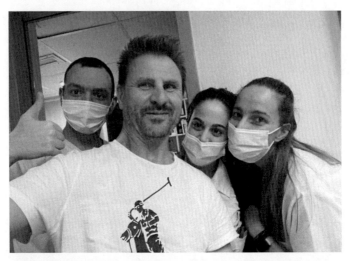

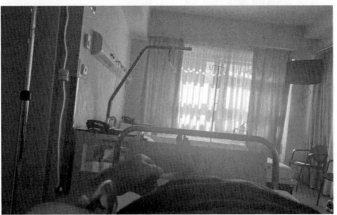

## Thursday 13 October

Thursday was the big operation day and my second intraprostatic injection would be carried out around 1.30 pm. In total I had the following procedures planned:

- Urethra dilation (to widen urethra and increase urine flow).

- Fibrinolytic agent injection (to stimulate tissue repair in the penis).

- Intraprostatic injection (to target the remaining bacteria and inflammation in my lower prostate near the connection with my urethra).

  The complete mixture of antibiotics that would be injected into my prostate was Tygacil, Meronem, Mefoxil, Voncon, Zithromax, Ciproxin and Zyvoxid.

- PRP penis injection (to stimulate blood flow and vessels in the penile shaft).

- PRP prostate injection (to help with increased prostate healing).

All of the procedures were expertly carried out under the Dr Pavlos's supervision while I was under general anaesthetic.

I woke up out of my daze to be in the pre-surgery room surrounded by some of the team of six people who were present during my surgery. The staff waited for me to be coherent enough to go back to the general intravenous therapy ward to rest and recuperate. This time I waited one hour before taking the bandage out of my anus. This was a good decision as there was less liquid and mess on this, my second intraprostatic procedure. I was able to rest for a while before visiting the doctor in the afternoon for a single PiezoWave prostate treatment, given no massage was permitted on the prostate after the injection.

After four more hours of IV antibiotics at The Central Clinic of Athens I was relieved to be back at my hotel after my tiring day of procedures starting at 7.30 am and finishing at 11 pm.

One thing I did differently on my second IV antibiotics/intraprostatic injection week was keep the cannula in my arm. This meant I didn't have to go through a nurse injecting a new vein every morning and it made the week somewhat easier to bear.

*I found keeping my cannula in was better than a nurse having to find a new vein to inject each day. Moving forward, if I had a comfortable injection wrapping, I was going to keep it in place during treatment week.*

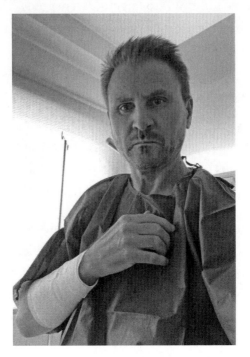

## Friday 14 October

When I woke up on the Friday morning after my prostate injection I was really tired. The strong mixture of antibiotics swirling through my system and the long week were taking a toll. It took real motivation to drag myself out of bed for three more hours of intravenous antibiotics from 8 am. I now had only two more three-hour IV antibiotic sessions and three more treatments with the doctor before my week was over and I was free again.

The urethra dilation during week seven of the program delivered a significant improvement in my urinary performance in just a few days.

*The charts below compare the Tuesday before the surgery (top – 17.4 ml/s maximum flow) to the Saturday after the surgery (bottom – 28.3 ml/s maximum flow).*

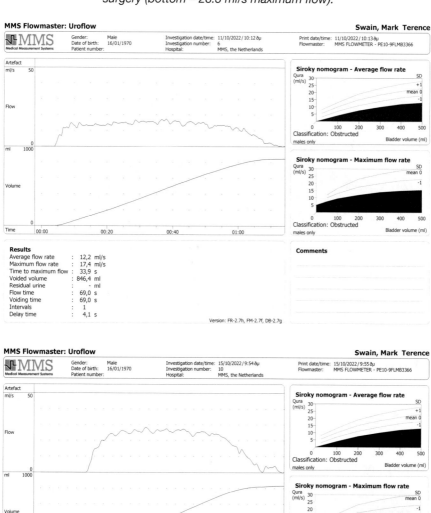

On the Saturday morning I paid the Athens Clinic accounting department €1000 for my hospital stay and antibiotics. Then I was off in a taxi to the beachside suburb of Glyfada.

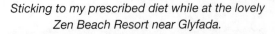

*Sticking to my prescribed diet while at the lovely Zen Beach Resort near Glyfada.*

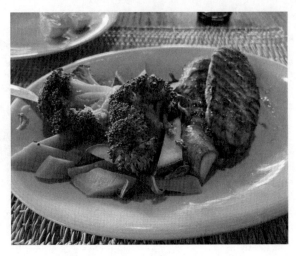

## WEEK 7: Continued prostate treatment and antibiotic reduction and provision of additional vitamins and probiotics to support the body.
### *The toughest week so far.*

### Monday 17 October

I came back to the seventh week of treatment tired and cranky after two interrupted nights of sleep at the Azur Suites, Glyfada. It was a nice weekend getaway to a beautiful beach and cosmopolitan area only thirty minutes out of Athens. However, it made me realise how important good sleep is on this program (it's obviously important at all times, but even more so when your immune system is fighting harmful bacteria). My choice of accommodation near a road was not a good one and I could hear horns beeping, trucks revving and loud motorbikes most of the night.

I vowed I would never book my weekend relaxation accommodation near a road or any noise again. My weekend really did come to a shuddering halt as I arrived in Athens at 10.30 am for my first prostate massage of the week and first since my prostate injection last Thursday. My prostate felt sensitive to touch, but luckily the doctor was gentle on me again.

## It was feeling by now that my prostate was saying 'leave me alone'.

I was so low on energy as I had my morning prostate massage, prostate PiezoWave and penis PiezoWave treatment.

When I exited the clinic treatment room, I met another Aussie, Paul, who had just flown in to see Pavlos. I gave him some reassurances about the program and explained he was in good hands. We exchanged numbers and agreed to meet for a chat and bite to eat later. After this I left the clinic and went straight to my hotel room to lie down.

I didn't even have the energy to leave my hotel and get lunch. I just had some fruit in my room and rested most of the afternoon. The afternoon nap really did me good and I was reluctantly able to drag my backside out of bed and turn up for my 5.30 pm treatment.

*I've mentioned before that commitment is one of the three key factors in this program, alongside time and money. It's turning up on days like this when you really don't want to that are critical to the program's success.*

I took a mindset of breaking the program down into one day at a time. It was as if I was turning up to work every day. Sometimes I even took the program one second at a time, for instance when I was going through the prostate massage treatment. My attitude was just keep turning up and keep grinding through the program.

After my 5.30 pm treatment of another prostate massage and prostate PiezoWave, I caught up with fellow Australian Paul, whom I had met in the clinic earlier. We met for a light bite at Kavlo

Wnuevo Slovaki, very close to the doctor's clinic and The Central Clinic of Athens where the IV antibiotics are administered.

At only twenty-five years old Paul told me his story of how he had been really struggling with Chronic Prostatitis for three years. Like myself he had visited numerous specialists in Australia who all told him he was okay. Paul had visited as many as twenty urologists, most of which just gave him antibiotics and said his urinary and erection problems would clear up.

I felt sorry for such a young guy, who at twenty-five was being ravaged by the terror of Chronic Prostatitis. Paul mentioned how he had stopped going out with his friends and had become very antisocial. He also talked about in his desperation to get better, how he was self-administering antibiotics and trying different antibiotic mixes that he felt might cure the disease.

It was conversations with people like Paul and others who were really struggling that made me decide to share my story in this book.

## Tuesday 18 October

This was the toughest day of the program so far for me. It was my thirty-eighth day of treatment and I was moving into week seven of the program.

When I arrived at the clinic, I was tired enough to sleep on the floor. I felt as if my body was at the limits of what it could take. Maybe the constant treatment for over six weeks was starting to take its toll?

I explained to the doctor's wife Elena (who managed reception and administration) upon arrival that I was really struggling today, especially with lethargy and tiredness. Elena reassured me that it was normal during the program to have highs and lows. It was particularly normal to have a severe low the week after all the intra-venous antibiotics, she advised me. Elena mentioned she had seen this many times with other patients. Her supportive message was I would feel much stronger in two days. I hoped she was right.

When I met the doctor for my morning treatment, I also advised him I was really struggling.

## Now, I'm not a quitter, but this was the closest I had come to quitting the program.

Pavlos mentioned the antibiotics used in the intravenous treatment last week were very strong and it was perfectly normal for the body to have this reaction. He immediately cut back my daily antibiotic Norocin and prescribed some Lamberts Multi-Guard high-strength vitamins. I was also taking omega 3, liver refresh, colostrum and probiotic tablets at this stage to counteract all the antibiotics I was taking and to maintain a healthy immune and digestive system. The probiotics in particular were very important to provide additional support for the body while the antibiotics were being taken.

I proceeded to have my regular morning treatment of prostate massage, prostate PiezoWaves and penis PiezoWaves. This session was a real struggle to get through due to my prostate feeling sensitive and my really bad tiredness and lethargy. I walked out of the session with my legs barely able to carry me.

Again, I was struggling to go to lunch at my daily lunch spot, Nikitas. Nikitas served home-cooked, nutritious food that really helped me get through the program. Panos and the team there couldn't have done any more to support my rejuvenation journey with their daily healthy special menu and home-cooked food. But I did motivate myself to go to Nikitas and was very pleased I did. The lentil soup and roast chicken with vegetables was delicious; everything I needed to help get my drained energy back.

The afternoon was my regular siesta at the Dunlin Hotel before heading out for treatment two of the day at 5.30 pm.

By now I had got to meet many other patients going through a similar rejuvenation journey to mine. Christos, Lukas, Efy, Dimos, Alexis, Ellie and more were always supportive, and we often had some real banter and jokes in the doctor's reception. It was always nice to speak to other patients and hear how their unique treatment and recovery programs were progressing.

After my 5.30 pm massage and PiezoWave treatment I'd done it – I'd gotten through the toughest day of the program so far. I went back to my hotel and crashed.

## Wednesday 19 October

Thankfully I woke up feeling much less tired than yesterday. I was able to take my first Lamberts Multi-Guard vitamins on an empty stomach first thing in the morning, and restarted some Intelecta Levocarnitine to help further boost my immune system. My body had essentially been weakened by all the strong antibiotics I had taken last week.

It was then my normal twenty-minute walk to the clinic again after my now go-to breakfast of boiled egg, avocado, spinach and one slice of rye bread.

*When I was struggling in week seven of the program following my second intraprostatic injection, I started taking daily Intelecta Levocarnitine and Lamberts Multi-Guard high-strength vitamins to boost my immune system.*

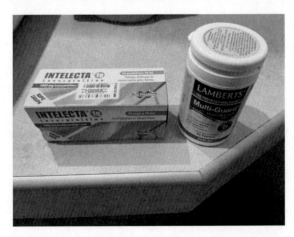

Today and for the rest of the week up to and including Saturday morning I did my regular daily treatment program.

## Morning

- Prostate massage (one minute × four)
- Prostate PiezoWave (ten minutes)
- Sexual dysfunction penis erection PiezoWave treatment (fifteen minutes)

## Evening

- Prostate massage (one minute × four)
- Prostate PiezoWave (ten minutes)

While the prostate massages were never something to look forward to, they were now not nearly as bad as the first few days. I was now actually starting to notice my prostate felt much softer and more comfortable to touch.

After getting through this, the toughest week, I was delighted to be heading out of busy Athens again to relax in the suburban beachside area of Voula.

*Following the doctor's orders by relaxing and eating well at Zen Beach, thirty minutes out of Athens. I had made it through week seven, the toughest of the program for me.*

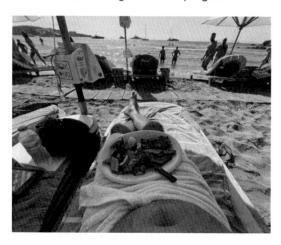

I also think this week was a struggle because I had originally planned and prepared to be in Athens for a six-week treatment program. I was psychologically preparing to leave a week ago, but because the doctor had found additional complications with me in sexual dysfunction and urinary stricture of the urethra, I now needed to stay for ten weeks.

## WEEK 8: Further elimination of prostate inflammation. Attacking the central part of early infection. Further sexual dysfunction treatment.

As my inflammation in the prostate was reducing, it was now time to start tackling the most long-standing central part of the infection, the infection that had built up over the longest amount of time.

I'd had fantastic rest and sleep at Zen Beach and Voula over the weekend, with the ocean swims and sunshine doing me the world of good. The fact I was the only person in Molly Malone's Irish bar on Saturday evening in Glyfada drinking Chamomile tea while watching the English Premiership football made me look a little bit weird, but hey, who cares if I was getting better!

### Monday 24 October

I was back in the clinic at 10.30 Monday morning to start week eight of the program. This was the best I was looking and feeling in the program so far.

*Looking leaner and meaner at Zen Beach on Sunday
23 October 2022. I'd gone from 78.5 kg to 73 kg since the
start of the program on 5 September 2022.*

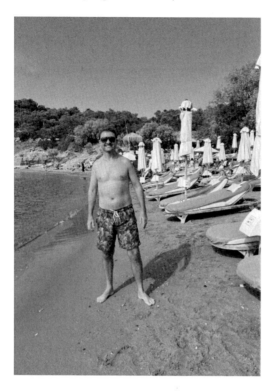

Other patients were starting to tell me how I was looking younger every day. People would mention that my skin looked better and my eyes were cleaner, with no dark bags underneath them. Maybe the prostate massages and diet were working after all?

Pavlos completed his normal treatment on me Monday morning and Monday early evening.

## Morning

- Prostate massage (one minute × four)
- Prostate PiezoWave (ten minutes)
- Sexual dysfunction penis erection PiezoWave treatment (fifteen minutes)

## Evening

- Prostate massage (one minute × four)
- Prostate PiezoWave (ten minutes)

During the week I was 100% focused on getting through the treatment program each day and doing everything I could to support my recovery. My daily focus was to:

- sleep well
- get through the treatment
- eat healthily
- not over-exert my body (I only did walks and weekend ocean swims as exercise)
- cut social media and stress out of my life
- read and relax more.

Both Elena and Pavlos at the clinic had constantly told me that the patients with the most positive outlook and approach to recovery make the fastest progress.

I met some patients who thought they could still eat kebabs with fries and white pita bread. You simply cannot do this on the program. You cannot sneak in a quick beer or piece of sugary cake. This just gives the infecting microbes an environment to regroup and thrive again. (The microbes in particular love feeding on sugar, which as we all know is in most sweet treats and 'naughty' foods.)

I did my normal treatment through Monday, Tuesday and Wednesday.

## Thursday 27 October

I had a stiff neck during the night, and also woke up with a stiff neck and stiff upper mid back. I didn't know whether this was part of me getting better or my body changing and adapting. It was certainly noticeable through this week how my body stiffness escalated.

I'd had these symptoms before but not while in the treatment period. I also felt like my ears were starting to block again. I actually felt a bit more demoralised preparing to have my first treatment. I felt like I had taken a couple of steps backwards. I thought maybe it was just another low as part of the recovery process after my high of yesterday when I was feeling great.

I headed off to my 9.30 appointment on Thursday morning with a stiff neck, stiff shoulders and stiff back. I also had some pain in my left flank for good measure. The joys of Chronic Prostatitis!

During my morning meeting with the doctor, I explained how I was struggling with a stiff neck and back. He explained that the microbes in the prostate cause strangulation of nerves, which often affect the back and neck. The pain was more pronounced that day because I had cut back to only one antibiotic a day, Ceftoral, due to my body's fatigue after my last intravenous treatment. The decision to cut back to one antibiotic a day and ditch the twice-daily Norocin was based on how tired my body was last week after intravenous week two.

The doctor prescribed another stronger antibiotic, Augmentin, to subdue the neck pain and stiffness.

One of the key benefits of the Georgiadis Treatment Protocol is the doctor is always listening to how you are feeling during your daily appointments. This allows him to continually modify the treatment and medicine mix for maximum patient benefit.

While I was having my prostate electrification session, pulses could be felt in my right ear. This showed me how the prostate and its strangulation was so connected right up through the body up to my brain and ears. This strangulation was also causing my neck and back pain.

In simple terms, the reason the back pain had surfaced was my antibiotics had been reduced. Any microbes that were left in the prostate could more easily group and cause strangulation as they had less antibiotics to fight.

I left the surgery on Thursday to grab a coffee and stock up on my new antibiotics, Augmentin, at the friendly pharmacy down the road.

After lunch, this was the second day on the program that I did not need a siesta to rest (a very encouraging sign). I was starting to not be so tired and drained after my morning, and indeed evening, prostate massages.

On the Thursday of week eight I had a real spring in my step as I walked to my 8 pm appointment. I had been singing and dancing in my hotel room before leaving and just felt so happy. It was a wonderful sign for me and I felt like I was getting my old life back. I cannot even explain where the sudden burst of energy came from; I just felt positive and happy.

*The pharmacy where I got all my antibiotics in Athens. This is very close to the doctor's clinic and The Central Clinic of Athens where intraprostatic injections are carried out. It also had a set of scales I would regularly weigh myself on to monitor my weight reduction.*

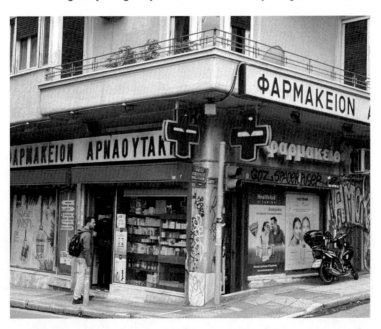

The doctor was pleased to hear I was feeling happy and lively. He said it was the new antibiotic Augmentin attacking the microbes that often make people feel tired and melancholic.

The evening prostate massage and prostate PiezoWave were easy to manage today and I walked home in a relaxed and positive state. When I went to bed I had much less pain in my neck and shoulders.

## Friday 28 October

I woke up at 4 am on the Friday and could feel the new antibiotic Augmentin working. Things were happening in my body. The weird wriggling sensation in my ears came back, but this time it felt like it was more of a contracting feeling. It was like the small things or microbes causing wriggling in my ear were getting smaller.

I was also getting wave sensations rolling down the back of my neck which was like my body trying to cure the neck stiffness. It was starting to feel like the new antibiotic Augmentin was working on me in varied and mysterious ways, all of which seemed to be positive and healing.

Again, this highlights how much problems with your prostate affect your sensory feelings and nerves all the way up through your body and down through your legs.

One thing that astounded me about Chronic Prostatitis is how it affects so many far-reaching parts of your body. For me, the nerve strangulation caused swelling in my brain, blocking in my ears, lost sensation in my right thigh, lower back pain, left flank pain and tingling in my right foot.

After my treatment, I caught up with fellow patient Dimos for lunch and to hear his story and journey fighting Chronic Prostatitis. (His case study is included in part III, alongside others).

By this stage of the program, having nearly completed week eight, I felt as follows:

## Progress

- My mind felt sharper.
- I was happier and more positive.
- I needed to urinate less frequently.
- My urine flow was better.
- I didn't feel so tired when I woke up.
- My erections were stronger and more regular.

## Concerns

- I still had pain in my neck and back.
- Occasionally I still had the blocking sensation in my ears.
- Sometimes (less frequently) I still had the tingling sensation in my penis causing the need to urinate.
- Intermittent pain in my left flank.

Overall, though, by now I was feeling and looking much better; this was also the third day in a row I did not need a siesta.

On the last morning of week eight while relaxing in my hotel room before my Saturday morning treatment I had the craziest itching sensation in my right ear for two minutes or so. I felt like I needed to insert something into my ear and scratch it. This was a sensation I used to get regularly at the peak of my symptoms, and it was the first time I'd had it in the ten weeks of the program. Upon meeting the doctor on the Saturday morning, he advised me the wriggling sensation in my ears was the auditory nerves being affected by reflective messaging from the prostate.

After my prostate massage this morning the doctor asked me if my ears were still ringing and itching. Given he had done a stronger prostate massage than normal, I said to him in humour let me worry about getting my breath back first!

Essentially nerves that the prostate strangulates and traps have a reflective capability to then affect other nerves. Pavlos also told me that he'd had patients who'd had their spine operated on when it was not even necessary. Getting rid of the strangulation and sclerotic tissue in the prostate would have gotten rid of their back pain rather than a costly and unnecessary back operation on a patient who didn't even need it.

The eighth week of treatment was now complete and I was able to head off straight to Zen Beach again to relax. I needed to recharge my batteries for next week's third intensive intravenous antibiotics week and third intraprostatic injection.

## WEEK 9: Third injection in the prostate to specifically target small long-standing spots of infection. Attacking the core.

### Monday 31 October

This would be the week of my third intraprostatic injection. After my relaxing weekend in Voula, some twenty-five minutes outside of Athens, I took a taxi back to Central Athens to start the week's treatment.

I noticed on the way back I had symptoms of stiff shoulders, neck and back. This was surprising to me as I really slept and rested well over the weekend. I also had a mildly itchy anus when I woke up, which demonstrated to me the microbes in my body were still doing some nasty work.

I went straight to The Central Clinic of Athens to do my COVID-19 PCR test to confirm I was safe to enter the clinic the next day and start my IV antibiotic treatment. Once again, my drip antibiotics would be starting on Tuesday.

The daily treatment of a prostate massage, prostate PiezoWave and penis PiezoWave for sexual dysfunction was pretty easy to get through. I was free to now check back into the Dunlin Hotel and grab lunch at the always-friendly and delicious Nikitas.

After lunch I felt pretty tired and had an aching neck and back, so I went to my hotel for a siesta before Monday's treatment two. I really felt like I needed a siesta, which for me was common throughout the treatment program as my body processed the toxins that were flushed out during the morning prostate massages.

In the afternoon the doctor's surgery was very busy as new patients arrived from around the world. I had a nice chat with Christian from the UK who had been experiencing urination problems for years and had totally lost his sex drive.

My evening prostate massage went fine, and actually my prostate felt very smooth when the doctor touched it (over time the prostate massages thankfully became easier and less painful). My prostate PiezoWave treatment was business as usual and I was out of the clinic at 8 pm, ready to eat and rest up for the IV antibiotic days ahead.

## Tuesday 1 November

I woke up feeling pretty tired and groggy, with an aching neck and back again. It felt like I was coming down with the flu but it was surely just more Chronic Prostatitis symptoms. It took effort and determination to roll out of bed and head to The Central Clinic of Athens for three hours of IV antibiotics on intravenous day one.

Following this, on the Tuesday I completed my now regular morning treatment routine of:

### Morning

- Prostate massage (one minute × four)
- Prostate PiezoWave (ten minutes)
- Sexual dysfunction penis erection PiezoWave treatment (fifteen minutes)

In the afternoon the doctor performed the third transrectal ultrasound on my prostate and eleventh uroflow test on my urination, to test my vital statistics pre-surgery.

*My third prostate scan showed much reduced inflammation and a prostate that had reduced to 11.28 ml from the original 15.02 ml.*

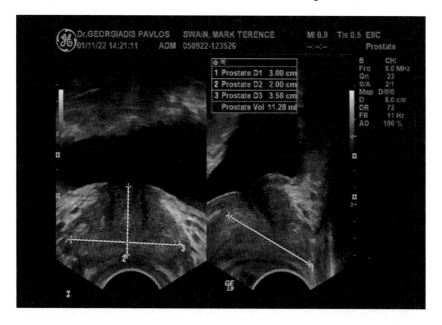

*My eleventh uroflow test showed a marked improvement. The urination flow was now looking even more like a bell curve compared to the original uroflow test taken at the start of my treatment.*

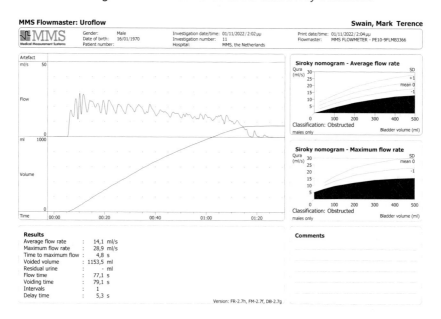

In the afternoon I had my second prostate massage of the day and second prostate PiezoWave treatment. They both went smoothly, and it was time to head to the hotel and rest to prepare for more intravenous antibiotics the next day.

## Wednesday 2 November

This was the day before my intraprostatic surgery. I was at The Central Clinic of Athens by 8 am to start my IV antibiotics over the next two-and-a-half hours.

I had not finished all my antibiotics when the doctor texted me to come and have my regular morning treatment of prostate massage, prostate PiezoWave and penis PiezoWave. I then headed back to the IV treatment room to finish my morning IV antibiotics with a fusilli wholegrain pasta and vegetable meal from Cultivos cafe in hand, which I ate in the treatment room. It was a long morning and I departed from the morning's treatment and antibiotics at 2 pm.

At 5.30 I was back in the doctor's surgery for my regular evening treatment of:

### Evening

- Prostate massage (one minute × four)
- Prostate PiezoWave (ten minutes)

After this I had two more hours of IV antibiotics at the clinic with 250 ml of Voncon, 100 ml of Meronem, 300 ml of Zyvoxid and 4 ml of Zofran slowly dripping into me before surgery the next day.

## Thursday 3 November

Surgery day is always a big, demanding day, I had come to learn. I had a very light breakfast of half an avocado, two boiled eggs (one without yolk, to keep the carbohydrates low) and half a slice of rye bread with two small glasses of water at 7 am. It is recommended to have no or a very light breakfast the day of intraprostatic injection surgery.

My intravenous antibiotics started at 8.30 am for two-and-a-half hours before I went to the doctor for a prostate massage, prostate PiezoWave and penis PiezoWave treatment. The prostate massage was much stronger today as the doctor wanted to disturb any microbes hiding out in my prostate sclerotic tissue. After the treatment I was back to the clinic to finish two more bottles of the morning's antibiotics.

By 1.30 pm there was still a bottle to go, but it was time for surgery. A nurse appeared with urgency and asked me to change into the now familiar operating gown, plastic socks and hospital-style underwear. What a sight I was again!

I walked down to the operating theatre this time to be greeted by the team of six or seven doctors and nurses and Pavlos, who would be coordinating proceedings.

Quickly a liquid was entering my arm via IV and I went dozy before drifting off into the clouds. I awoke with all the injections done, including a PRP on the penis to enhance the healing process, plus my third intraprostatic injection. I was wheeled back on a hospital bed to the IV ward where I finished my last bottle of the morning's antibiotics at 4.30 pm.

I was absolutely starving by now as I hadn't eaten since my light breakfast. I quickly demolished a Greek salad and grilled salmon skewers at my go-to souvlaki restaurant.

I didn't even have time to go back to my hotel room to rest. It was another prostate PiezoWave treatment at 6.30 pm before more IV antibiotics between 7 pm and 10.30 pm.

I walked back to the hotel gingerly, tired after a non-stop medical day that started at 8.30 am.

## Friday 4 November

Following yesterday's intraprostatic injection, more IV treatment followed between 8.30 and 10.45 am, 11.45 am and 1 pm and 7 and 10.30 pm.

I didn't have a prostate massage as it was still sensitive after the injection. The intraprostatic injection is specifically designed to target the remaining areas where there is inflammation and infection. I felt the doctor had really hit the bullseye on my prostate inflammation the previous day as I had a sharp left-flank pain.

Between 11 and 11.45 am I had a prostate PiezoWave and penis PiezoWave treatment.

By this third week of IV antibiotics and third intraprostatic injection I was starting to get very familiar with the procedure.

## At this stage of the program I was noticing having erections so much more frequently.

I didn't sleep as well on the Friday night after surgery as the cannula was still in my arm and I awoke about every two hours. Whenever I woke up, I had a raging erection. Whatever Pavlos was doing seemed to be working down below!

### Saturday 5 November

I mentioned the ridiculously regular erections I was getting to the doctor on the Saturday morning and his comment was, 'Bravo, that's excellent'. That was good enough for me.

On Saturday morning I did my final two-and-a-half hours of intravenous antibiotics between 8.30 and 11.00 am before heading to the doctor's clinic for a prostate PiezoWave and penis PiezoWave. I then completed my final IV antibiotics for the week between 12 and 1 pm. I quickly paid my €1000 hospital bill for the week before jumping in a taxi to relax at my now regular retreat in Voula.

I was tired and jaded, but I had gotten through my third injection week. I was really glad to have ground my way through another IV week, knowing the treatment was ultimately doing me good and getting my life back.

I was really tired after this, my third prostate injection week, and headed straight to Zen Beach for their delicious fish soup and grilled chicken with vegetables. By 4 pm I just needed to sleep so I had a two-hour siesta. I then slept the whole night from 8.30 pm to 7.30 am, only waking a couple of times with my now all too familiar erections.

One additional thing I noticed that weekend was I was now chewing on the left side of my jaw and mouth while eating.

> It seems Chronic Prostatitis had even affected my jaw and stopped me chewing on the left side.

This was another one of the many weird symptoms of Chronic Prostatitis I noticed as I was starting to heal.

## WEEK 10: Detailed prostate massages targeting final inflammation areas. Continual erectile treatment.

This was the last week of the program before I was given a two-week break from the antibiotics and daily treatments. I was being given a break to see how my body responded without any medicine. In addition, this would allow for a second sperm test when I returned free from antibiotics.

> Some of my writing may seem repetitive in describing the treatment, but I want to share with you the full story of exactly what I went through.

The simple fact is the treatment program is repetitive. It is a daily grind and requires great commitment, time and determination.

## Monday 7 November

I'd had another relaxing weekend in Voula to recharge my batteries. At 9.30 am I took a taxi back to Central Athens for another appointment with the doctor. Again, I was tired and lethargic for my 10.15 Monday morning appointment following last week's intravenous antibiotics. It was a common theme for me to be very tired after the big intravenous antibiotics week.

The previous night I noticed very strong erections every time I woke up. Pavlos explained to me that this was a very good sign and showed a healthy body, strong heart and good blood vessels.

The morning's prostate massage was fine. I felt a bit sensitive today from last week's injection but it was not painful. The dual PiezoWave treatment on my prostate and penis were uneventful. Another morning's treatment was ticked off and it was time for my morning coffee with almond milk (a lower fat and healthier option than normal milk) at Cultivos.

After lunch and a short rest, I was back for my 6 pm session. The prostate massage and prostate PiezoWave treatment were over in twenty minutes and I was free to relax.

## Tuesday 8 November

I mentioned to the doctor this morning that by now I was needing to urinate much less frequently during the day and not at all at night.

> Prior to starting the program, I would often need to urinate urgently and frequently. I would maybe urinate twenty times a day and once or twice at night.

This had reduced over 60%. Pavlos explained that it was another example of how Chronic Prostatitis slowly caused problems with your urinary system that you did not really notice. Your body adapted to the slow onset of issues, and often you just told yourself, 'Well, I am getting older!'

My morning three regular sets of treatment were done without issues. I left the clinic a bit tired from the treatment and went to my hotel to relax. Lunch and a siesta soon passed and I was back for my 7 pm appointment.

During my second prostate massage of the day the doctor said my prostate was now in really good shape. He commented that I was following the program diligently and doing everything he asked of me. I had focused so hard on maintaining a healthy diet and relaxed mental state since the program started.

My prostate was feeling much softer and spongy by now, not like the hard stone prostate I walked in with nine-and-a-bit weeks ago. The PiezoWave was easy and painless, and after some brief banter with fellow patients Efy, Stratos and Dimos, I headed to the hotel to eat and relax.

## Wednesday 9 November

Today was the day for another uroflow urination (number twelve) before my regular treatment. The uroflow test is designed to measure how well urine is flowing and if the urethra is restricted by inflammation or sclerotic tissue in any way.

The second chart shows that my maximum flow was much higher and the overall shape shows a much smoother urination. This shows there is less strain on the bladder due to less inflammation.

The doctor was very happy with my improved urinary performance. I was also very happy as it was another clear visual example that I was improving and recovering from Chronic Prostatitis.

For me, one of the highlights of the treatment program was constantly seeing visible scientific evidence I was improving.

After my uroflow test I had my regular prostate massage, prostate PiezoWave and PiezoWave treatment for sexual dysfunction.

I caught up with fellow patient Dimos afterwards to compare our latest urination uroflow charts. This is one thing I never expected to do with another male in my life! It's actually surprising how quickly you become comfortable talking to fellow patients about your specific treatment plan and progress. While it is a very private matter, you all soon realise you are in the same boat fighting Chronic Prostatitis and wanting to get your life back.

I didn't feel tired so no time was needed for a siesta. This for me was a significant improvement – my tiredness and lethargy were reducing. I did some more work on this book with my new energetic and productive mindset.

I had some great banter with fellow patients Efy, Dimos and Christian prior to my 7 pm appointment. My prostate massage from Pavlos was strong but generally painless.

## The pain during the prostate massages had significantly reduced over time as my sclerotic tissue had been broken down.

Pavlos and I talked about how his treatment methodology is unique and obviously works. I'd started by now to research more for writing this book and I could not believe what rubbish was out there about Chronic Prostatitis. Some people were recommending listening to Beethoven, fingering your own prostate and applying bees' pollen to the prostate as cures. Even if these strange concepts did work (which they don't), I knew I could only successfully perform one of the three. I will let you guess which one that is …

*My original uroflow on the 5 September (top) compared to my twelfth
uroflow on the 9 November (bottom) showed a marked improvement.*

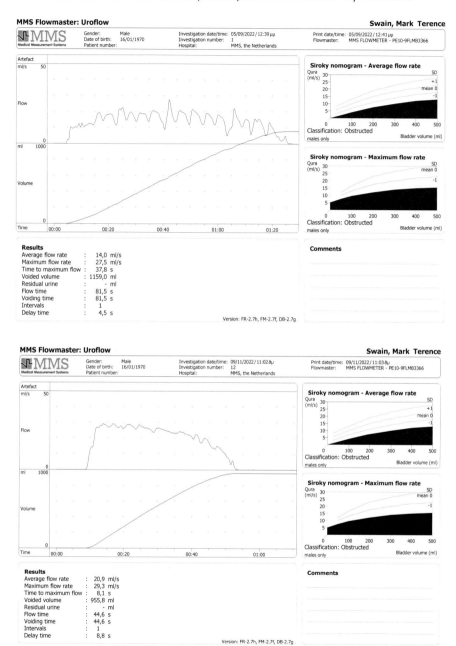

## Thursday 10 November

Between 11.00 and 11.45 am my normal morning treatment was carried out:

### Morning

- Prostate massage (one minute × four)
- Prostate PiezoWave (ten minutes)
- Sexual dysfunction penis erection PiezoWave treatment (fifteen minutes)

I had a great chat while waiting for my morning appointment with Jarrod from the US, who like me had done an intense nine-week program in Athens three months ago.

He explained how he was feeling much better and his inflammation was 99% clear now. We agreed to catch up for a coffee the next day as he was off to the Mycolab Laboratory to submit a sperm sample. The sperm test is done after some time away from the program with no antibiotics. It is designed to measure how much the microbes and bacteria have reduced during the treatment program so far.

In the evening I completed my regular session of a prostate massage and prostate PiezoWave.

I now had only one-and-a-half days to go now before I got a two-week break from the program. To say I was happy was an understatement.

## Friday 11 November

It was another pleasant sunny morning in Athens. I had a lovely stroll in the late summer sun to the doctor's clinic for my 10.30 am appointment.

The doctor mentioned again that my prostate was in good shape; it was now about breaking down the final details of the inflammation, which he advised was very important.

The prostate PiezoWave was as easy as normal and I nearly fell asleep during it for the first time. The sexual dysfunction device applied to give me an erection seemed to be put on turbocharge today and it gave my right ear a flickering sensation as I reached maximum hardness.

For me this continued to show how intricately the penis and prostate are linked to the ears as well as other places. My right ear had felt like a problem spot for me for a long time and I was beginning to see why.

I caught up with fellow patient Dimos for a coffee after treatment. He told me one story he had heard in the clinic from another patient.

This patient had complained of testicle pain. His local doctor advised it was because his testicles were banging together during sexual intercourse.

Now I know there are some terrible misdiagnoses regarding Chronic Prostatitis, but if you have heard a worse one than this, please email me at mark@chronicprostatits.org. I'd love to hear it.

Dimos also told me how some men who could not produce babies with their partners due to Chronic Prostatitis were after their treatment able to get their partners pregnant. These men would send photos of their new babies to the doctor, who would shed a tear of happiness for them.

Pavlos told me I should get some condoms for my future sexual activity. This would avoid sharing or contracting any microbes with my partner. I dutifully crossed the road to the supermarket after my treatment, and there was a priest standing right next to the condoms. What message was this trying to give me?

*I'm advised to buy condoms for my future sexual activity.*
*There was a priest right next to the condoms in the supermarket.*

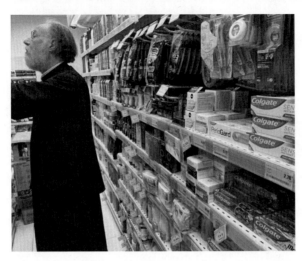

This freaked me out and I left the supermarket without purchasing any condoms. I vowed to return later and get some when the priest had – hopefully – gone.

After my lunch and a brief siesta, I got ready for my 6 pm treatment. There was lots of jokes and banter with fellow patients Jarrod, Ellie, Stratos, Dimos and Vassilis, given this was my last evening treatment for two weeks.

The evening prostate massage was very heavy. I think Pavlos wanted to massage me as hard as possible before my break. There was an easy PiezoWave treatment to follow to wrap up my last full day of treatment.

I then crossed the road to buy condoms – the priest had gone – before heading home for my last night in the Dunlin Hotel for a while.

## Saturday 12 November

I was up at 7 am to pack and get ready for departure today. My final morning session consisted of the usual program over 45 minutes.

**Morning**
- Prostate massage (one minute × four)
- Prostate PiezoWave (ten minutes)
- Sexual dysfunction penis erection treatment (twenty minutes)

During treatment I was chatting to Pavlos and I explained I'd had a really bad episode of COVID-19 over a six-week period prior to coming to Greece. He explained Chronic Prostatitis caused my immune system to be low which meant COVID-19 affected me much more than my friends who did not have Chronic Prostatitis. This made me even more determined to fully rid myself of this disease when I came back for more treatment in two weeks.

## Two weeks break from the program.
## All antibiotics stopped.

After my first ten weeks of intense Chronic Prostatitis treatment, I returned home to my mother's house in the UK for a two-week break. The antibiotics were stopped and I was free to rest and relax.

I could not believe how different and how much better I felt going back to the house I departed from on 1 September with Chronic Prostatitis just ten weeks ago. I woke up on the first day at my mother's house at 6.30 am feeling fresh and alive. This was a totally different feeling to when I was last there, where I always felt exhausted after a good night's sleep. I was able to do a nice thirty-minute morning walk and started typing up this book.

### I just felt so much more dynamic and proactive.

I continued with my healthy diet by having avocado, boiled eggs, spinach and a slice of rye bread for breakfast. This was followed by fruit, nuts and Greek yoghurt. I spent three hours on this book and was able to work with a clear head for the first time in a long time. I had a healthy poached salmon and vegetable lunch before visiting my Aunt and Uncle to tell them about my Athens medical treatment.

## Family members were simply stunned at how healthy and young I looked.

I was able to do another nice afternoon walk as my energy levels were much better.

The next day I was focused, sharp and productive again. It was a stark contrast to when I was last in England. I can honestly say I felt sixty-five years old when I left the UK and felt thirty-five years old when I returned after my first phase of Chronic Prostatitis treatment.

## Clear, focused, determined and calm seemed to be the words to describe me now.

On my third day back an old school friend visited me on the way home from his work. He was the same age as me at fifty-three but looked more like sixty. His body was worn out from years of neglect and his health seemed bad. This friend had a bad diet, low exercise levels, poor sleep, drank little water, and I'm convinced he also had Chronic Prostatitis due to his frequent night-time urination.

The doctor did say to me before departing Greece that my friends would now look so much older – he was right.

I continued my healthy diet and productive work during the rest of my first week off in the UK. I was getting regular strong erections in the night, and often ejaculated and had wet dreams.

My energy levels were just so much higher to exercise, do walks, generate productive work and complete odd jobs. Tasks that I would previously put off due to feeling lethargic and foggy headed were simply not an issue, and I tackled all tasks with gusto, usually immediately.

On my sixth night back, I went to visit a friend and his wife. We had a good discussion about her business ideas and plans. I was so much more engaged in the conversation than when I was previously there three months ago, and found it hard to believe how clear-headed, positive and fresh I felt.

My time off in the UK was followed by a week's golfing in Turkey. It was a revelation for me in terms of how I now felt and looked. My first phase of Chronic Prostatitis treatment had truly rejuvenated me and turned me into a more positive, dynamic and healthier person: the person I used to be before Chronic Prostatitis struck.

It was a challenge leaving the UK again after my two weeks break to go back to the treatment program in Athens. I can see how easy it is for patients to give up at this stage of the treatment if they are feeling so much better, with little or no symptoms. The challenge, however, is a limited number of microbes and small amounts of inflammation still exist; it is critical all of this is eliminated to fully eradicate Chronic Prostatitis long term.

## WEEK 11: Back to treatment. Second bacterial sperm test to measure progress in totally eliminating harmful bacteria causing Chronic Prostatitis.

### Tuesday 29 November

After my two weeks break, I was back to Athens to continue my treatment. I visited the doctor's clinic again at 11 am on Tuesday and Elena and Pavlos were pleased to see me again.

The first task was for me to have a transrectal scan to see how my prostate was currently looking. The results demonstrate how my prostate had further reduced in size.

The doctor explained he was very happy with my results, particularly the white healing of dark areas that were previously infected.

I then had my first prostate massage in two weeks. It was not painful, even though the doctor pressed hard to reach the centre of my remaining prostate infection and inflammation.

*My fourth prostate scan showed a further reduced size.*
*It was down to 10.47 ml from the original 15.02 ml.*

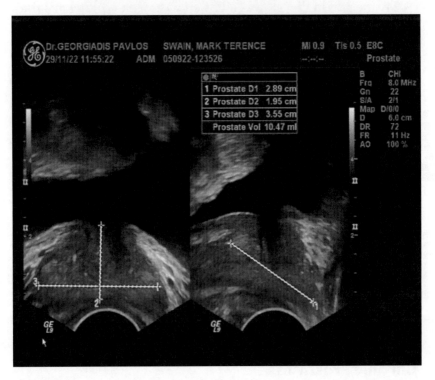

After my prostate massage I went to Mycolab (twenty minutes by taxi outside Athens centre) for my second sperm examination. I duly made my deposit in the now familiar dental-style room and the friendly employee advised me my results would be back in six to seven days. It was then time for a healthy lunch of lentil soup and broccoli salad at my regular go-to restaurant Nikitas, before heading to my hotel to relax.

In the early evening I visited the doctor's clinic again to perform my thirteenth uroflow test.

I also did a prostate PiezoWave to complete my first day back after the two-week break. It was also nice catching up with fellow patients Efy, Stratos, Nikolas and Christian again.

*My week-eleven uroflow test showed a stronger flow but a little less than the last test. This indicated inflammation was still present.*

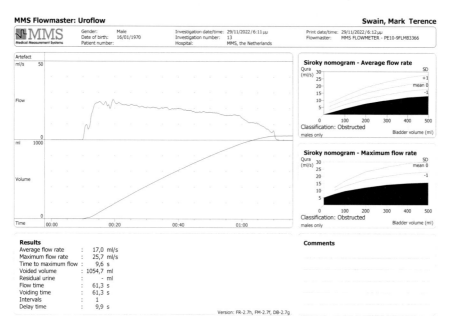

| MMS Flowmaster: Uroflow | | | | | Swain, Mark Terence |
|---|---|---|---|---|---|

**Results**

| | | |
|---|---|---|
| Average flow rate | : | 17,0 ml/s |
| Maximum flow rate | : | 25,7 ml/s |
| Time to maximum flow | : | 9,6 s |
| Voided volume | : | 1054,7 ml |
| Residual urine | : | - ml |
| Flow time | : | 61,3 s |
| Voiding time | : | 61,3 s |
| Intervals | : | 1 |
| Delay time | : | 9,9 s |

Version: FR-2.7h, FM-2.7f, DB-2.7g

**Comments**

## Wednesday 30 November

The weather was now much colder in Athens than when I was last there and I left my hotel in rainy and cold conditions for my 10.30 am appointment. Waterproof clothes were sometimes needed now as the weather had definitely changed from just two weeks ago.

The doctor put me back on my regular morning treatment program of:

### Morning

- Prostate massage (one minute × four)

- Prostate PiezoWave (ten minutes)
- Sexual dysfunction penis erection PiezoWave treatment (fifteen minutes)

The prostate massage was hard and stretched my anus quite a bit in order to press on the original central part of the infection and inflammation. The doctor's opinion was that I was now 80% better, hence I felt so much better during my two-week break.

The PiezoWave on my prostate was relaxed and painless as usual. The penis PiezoWave felt like it was penetrating my penis more deeply than before the break. The doctor advised this was because my penile tissue was healthier now and responded better to the regenerative shockwaves.

After my morning treatment I caught up with fellow patient and now friend Dimos for a coffee. It was great to hear and see his new positive mindset and how he was progressing so well with his treatment.

I had much more energy in the afternoon and did not need a siesta like I used to. I worked on this book in the afternoon and watched some World Cup Football.

I had a late prostate massage and PiezoWave at 9.30 pm before resting and relaxing in my room, however I felt some sensitivity in my right thigh after taking antibiotics late in the night.

## Thursday 1 December

I was a bit more tired today when waking as my oral tablet antibiotics I started when coming back to the program earlier this week started to kick in.

My 10.30 am prostate massage went okay, but my anus was hurting as I got back into the daily prostate massage routine. The PiezoWave prostate treatment was also fine and the erection PiezoWave treatment was good, except for a small cut that developed on my penis following yesterday's session.

Another visit had been ticked off the program and it was time for coffee and lunch with Dimos. Again, in the afternoon a siesta was not needed and I was able to work more on this book.

By now my energy was good throughout the day, which for me was a big step forward.

In the evening I did another prostate massage and prostate PiezoWave and walked at a fast pace back to the hotel. I now noticed I was walking faster with much more energy.

On my way home I stopped at the pharmacy to weigh myself.

I now weighed 71 kg. I had lost 7.5 kg since starting the program's healthy diet three months ago.

### Friday 2 December

I visited the doctor this morning who performed the three sets of treatment as usual on me:

### Morning

- Prostate massage (to break down sclerotic prostate tissue)
- Prostate PiezoWave (to target central areas of infection and inflammation in the prostate)
- Sexual dysfunction penis erection PiezoWave treatment

The appointment was at 11.30 am and took about forty-five minutes.

The doctor advised me that next week would be the same normal treatment program but the following week would be my fourth intraprostatic injection. He said he was going to make me work hard on some strong antibiotics over the coming weeks. I was not sure I wanted to hear that, but I trusted his judgment.

In the evening at 9 pm I had another prostate massage. The doctor went quite firmly across all corners and edges of my prostate to try to press out any remaining inflammation. The PiezoWave on my prostate was uneventful and I nearly fell asleep through it.

While walking to the hotel I noticed some type of release of my central abdominal muscles – it felt like my long-standing problems were steadily releasing.

## Saturday 3 December

My first week back on treatment was nearly over and at 9.15 am I completed my now familiar prostate massage, prostate PiezoWave and penis PiezoWave.

I noticed during my prostate PiezoWave some nerve sensitivity which indicated the central focal point of my inflammation may be breaking down. By now I also felt more nerve sensitivity in the left side of my penis during the shockwave treatment. This indicated that any penile urethra inflammation was also breaking down.

By 10 am I was finished and was able to head down the coast to Voula to relax.

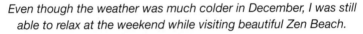

*Even though the weather was much colder in December, I was still able to relax at the weekend while visiting beautiful Zen Beach.*

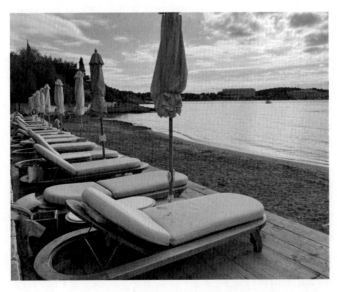

## WEEK 12: Further intense prostate massages and PiezoWave treatment to break down the most long-standing infected area.

On the Monday morning of week twelve I arrived from Voula back into the doctor's Athens clinic at 10.30 am. It was really busy this morning with some new patients arriving from the UK and US. While waiting, I had a good chat with new patients Chuck from the US and Adam from the UK. I reassured them they were in safe hands and gave them some tips to make their Greek stay a little more pleasant.

### It is somewhat daunting when you embark on your first detailed examination for Chronic Prostatitis.

My regular triple morning treatment of prostate massage, prostate PiezoWave and penis PiezoWave went without any problems.

In the evening I had a late 9.45 appointment, and during the prostate massage the long-standing hard bit in my prostate that previously hurt when massaged seemed to have disappeared. This final push to remove any residual inflammation and hard tissue seemed to be working.

I also felt much more sensitivity during the prostate PiezoWave up through my anus up into my prostate. The signals seemed to be more powerful, indicating more receptive nerves. It was another productive day of treatment and one more step closer to getting my life back.

### Tuesday 6 December

After working on this book more I went to a noon appointment with the doctor. He explained it was important to relay in this book that there is only one type of prostatitis and that is one caused by bacteria. Acute Prostatitis, Chronic Prostatitis and Pelvic Pain Syndrome are all essentially the same thing, he advised.

Prostatitis is always traced back to a single cause: microbial bacteria.

My prostate massage, prostate PiezoWave and penis PiezoWave went well. I was looking healthy and feeling good. Even at lunch the owner of Nikitas restaurant Panos said I was looking better and better each day. This was a big contrast to three months ago.

## Wednesday 7 December

My 11 am appointment of prostate massage, prostate PiezoWave and penis PiezoWave went without any issues. After my appointment I caught up with fellow patient Vaggelis, a fit 34-year-old capoeira instructor. His life had been decimated by Chronic Prostatitis (you can read his case study at the back of this book).

I did an evening prostate massage and prostate PiezoWave treatment at 9 pm. Before leaving the clinic, I spoke to patients Paul from Israel and Thomas from Greece to get their perspectives on what they would want to read in a book about Chronic Prostatitis.

## Thursday 8 December

I felt much more tired walking to my 11 am appointment. On arrival I explained to the doctor how I had low energy, felt tired and had a stiff neck. He asked that I immediately stop taking my twice-daily Augmentin antibiotic and Sporanox antifungal tablet. Both he explained can sometimes cause side effects of tiredness.

My prostate massage, prostate PiezoWave and penis PiezoWave were completed with no issues. It was time to grab a healthy lunch again.

While having lunch my email pinged with my second sperm test results from Mycolab.

I would later learn that cfu/ml is a colony-forming unit which estimates the number of viable bacteria in a sample that are able to multiply.

This new test clearly demonstrated that the program was working to reduce the bacterial microbes in my prostate. They had however not been fully eliminated.

After lunch and reading my results, I took my first siesta in a long time. My body seemed to need it today as it was struggling to adapt to all the antibiotics I was taking again. The siesta helped me pick up some energy and I was off to my 9 pm appointment.

The doctor said he had seen the results from my second sperm test and confirmed the microbes in my prostate had reduced significantly.

In total there was a 75% reduction in staphylococcus aureus and an 80% reduction in klebsiella pneumoniae bacteria.

The task ahead was now to fully eliminate these remaining microbes.

My 9 pm prostate massage and prostate PiezoWaves were painless and pretty easy to get through. I was ready to head to my hotel and rest up for tomorrow's two appointments with the doctor.

Upon walking home, I noticed the feeling in my right thigh start to come back. One of the symptoms Chronic Prostatitis had caused me was a numb right thigh. As I touched my thigh and gently hit it on the way home, it was evident feelings and a better sensation were coming back. Another good sign.

*My second sperm test showed that staphylococcus aureus and klebsiella pneumoniae were still present. The good news was staphylococcus aureus volumes had reduced from 80,000 cfu/ml to 20,000 cfu/ml and klebsiella pneumoniae had reduced from 100,000 cfu/ml to 20,000 cfu/ml.*

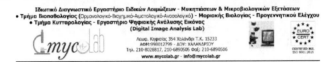

Ιδιωτικό Διαγνωστικό Εργαστήριο Ειδικών Λοιμώξεων - Μυκητιάσεων & Μικροβιολογικών Εξετάσεων
• Τμήμα Βιοπαθολογίας (Ορμονολογικό-Βιοχημικό-Αιματολογικό-Ανοσολογικό) - Μοριακής Βιολογίας - Προγεννητικού Ελέγχου
• Τμήμα Κυτταρολογίας - Εργαστήριο Ψηφιακής Ανάλυσης Εικόνας
(Digital Image Analysis Lab)

Λεωφ. Κηφισίας 354 Χαλάνδρι Τ.Κ. 15233
ΑΦΜ:998012799 - ΔΟΥ: ΧΑΛΑΝΔΡΙΟΥ
Τηλ. 210-8028817, 210-6890505 Φαξ: 210-6890506
www.mycolab.gr - info@mycolab.gr

## ANTIBIOGRAM

**MARK SWAIN**                              **Athens**        **29/11/2022**

Material :              *CULTURE OF SPERM*

Microbe :               *Staphylococcus aureus = 20.000  cfu/ml*

| | Classif/tion | MIC's | | Classif/tion | MIC's |
|---|---|---|---|---|---|
| PENICILLINE : | | | ERYTHROMYCIN: | R | |
| AMPICILLIN: | R | | CLARITHROMYCIN: | R | |
| AMOXICILLIN: | R | | ROXITHROMYCIN: | R | |
| AMOX.+AC.CLAVUL.: | S | | AZITHROMYCIN: | R | |
| AMPICIL.+SULBACT: | | | | | |
| PIPERACILLIN: | | | | | |
| PIPERACILLIN/TAZOBACTAM: | | | AZTREOENAM: | | |
| TICARCILLIN: | | | IMIPENEM: | | |
| TICARCILLIN+AC.CLAV.: | | | MEROPENEM: | | |
| | | | GENTAMICIN: | S | |
| | | | TOBRAMYCIN: | | |
| CEFADROXIL: | | | NETILMYCIN: | | |
| CEPHALOTHIN: | S | | AMICACIN: | S | |
| CEPHAZOLIN: | | | TETRACYCLIN: | R | |
| CEFAMANDOLE: | | | DOXYCYCLIN: | R | |
| CEFOXITINE: | S | | CLINDAMYCIN: | S | |
| CEFUROXIME SODIUM: | R | | METRONIDAZOLE: | | |
| CEFUROXIME AXETIL: | R | | CHLORAMPHENICOL: | S | |
| CEFACLOR: | | | TRIMETH. SULFA: | S | |
| CEFPROZIL: | | | NITROFURANTOIN: | S | |
| CEFIXIME: | R | | ACID FUSIDIC: | S | |

1 of 2

Pikro Software
210 6842098

Ιδιωτικό Διαγνωστικό Εργαστήριο Ειδικών Λοιμώξεων - Μυκητιάσεων & Μικροβιολογικών Εξετάσεων
• Τμήμα Βιοπαθολογίας (Ορμονολογικό-Βιοχημικό-Αιματολογικό-Ανοσολογικό) - Μοριακής Βιολογίας - Προγεννητικού Ελέγχου
• Τμήμα Κυτταρολογίας - Εργαστήριο Ψηφιακής Ανάλυσης Εικόνας
(Digital Image Analysis Lab)

Λεωφ. Κηφισίας 354 Χαλάνδρι Τ.Κ. 15233
ΑΦΜ:998012799 - ΔΟΥ: ΧΑΛΑΝΔΡΙΟΥ
Τηλ. 210-8028817, 210-6890505 Φαξ: 210-6890506
www.mycolab.gr - info@mycolab.gr

# ANTIBIOGRAM

**MARK SWAIN**                     **Athens**          **30/11/2022**

Material :        *CULTURE OF SPERM*

Microbe :        *Klebsiella pneumoniae = 20.000  cfu/ml*

| | Classif/tion | MIC's | | Classif/tion | MIC's |
|---|---|---|---|---|---|
| PENICILLINE : | | | ERYTHROMYCIN: | | |
| AMPICILLIN: | R | | CLARITHROMYCIN: | | |
| AMOXICILLIN: | R | | ROXITHROMYCIN: | R | |
| AMOX.+AC.CLAVUL.: | R | | AZITHROMYCIN: | R | |
| AMPICIL.+SULBACT: | | | | | |
| PIPERACILLIN: | S | | | | |
| PIPERACILLIN/TAZOBACTAM: | S | | AZTREOENAM: | S | |
| TICARCILLIN: | R | | IMIPENEM: | S | |
| TICARCILLIN+AC.CLAV.: | S | | MEROPENEM: | S | |
| | | | GENTAMICIN: | S | |
| | | | TOBRAMYCIN: | | |
| CEFADROXIL: | | | NETILMYCIN: | | |
| CEPHALOTHIN: | R | | AMICACIN: | S | |
| CEPHAZOLIN: | | | TETRACYCLIN: | S | |
| CEFAMANDOLE: | | | DOXYCYCLIN: | S | |
| CEFOXITINE: | S | | CLINDAMYCIN: | | |
| CEFUROXIME SODIUM: | S | | METRONIDAZOLE: | | |
| CEFUROXIME AXETIL: | S | | CHLORAMPHENICOL: | | |
| CEFACLOR: | S | | TRIMETH. SULFA: | S | |
| CEFPROZIL: | | | NITROFURANTOIN: | R | |
| CEFIXIME: | S | | ACID FUSIDIC: | R | |

1 of 2

## Friday 9 December

My appointment with the doctor was at 11.30 am and included my normal morning treatment of:

### Morning

- Prostate massage (one minute × four)
- Prostate PiezoWave (ten minutes)
- Sexual dysfunction penis erection PiezoWave treatment (fifteen minutes)

After my treatments, which took in total about forty-five minutes, I was free to eat, rest and relax ahead of my evening appointment.

My 8.30 pm appointment was uneventful and the prostate massage and prostate PiezoWave were easy to get through. I was even able to hang out with some fellow patients after my treatment, hear their Chronic Prostatitis stories and even take in some World Cup Football in the doctor's clinic.

## Saturday 10 December

My 9.45 am prostate massage, prostate PiezoWave and penis PiezoWave were over pretty easily this morning. I mentioned to the doctor that I'd had erections lots last night and he said, 'It is a sign everything is healing'.

I chatted to fellow patient Jarrod, who was off back to the US after completing a treatment program almost identical to mine. I promised to update him on how my next few weeks' treatment went.

I was now free to rest and relax at my weekend retreat in Voula. Next week would be my fourth intraprostatic injection and I would need all the energy I could muster to take on some very strong intravenous antibiotics.

## WEEK 13: Fourth intraprostatic injection to target final areas of infection and inflammation. Super strong intravenous antibiotics to try to eliminate the final bacteria.

This my thirteenth week of treatment would include five days of intravenous antibiotics and my fourth intraprostatic injection.

### Monday 12 December

My Monday morning started with a COVID-19 PCR test at The Central Clinic of Athens. This was to confirm I was safe to enter the hospital for treatment. Once my PCR test was done, I headed to the pharmacy to buy Bricklin, which would be injected into my prostate in three days.

The intravenous antibiotics ahead for the week were as follows:

### Morning (Tuesday and Wednesday)
- Voncon 250 ml
- Meronem 100 ml
- Zyvoxid 300 ml

### Evening (Tuesday and Wednesday)
- Voncon 250 ml
- Meronem 100 ml
- Zyvoxid 300 ml

### Morning (Thursday, Friday and Saturday)
- Voncon 250 ml
- Meronem 100 ml
- Tygacil 100 ml

### Evening (Thursday and Friday)
- Voncon 250 ml
- Meronem 100 ml
- Tygacil 100 ml

I completed my normal morning treatment of prostate massage, prostate PiezoWave and penis PiezoWave from 11.00 to 11.45 am. I was then free to have a latte with almond milk with fellow patient Dimos.

In the afternoon I rested after a healthy lunch of lentil soup, grilled veal and spinach, knowing a tough week was ahead.

In the evening I had my normal prostate massage and prostate PiezoWave. The doctor advised me I would have a uroflow test the next day and another transrectal prostate scan to measure my urine efficiency and any inflammation in my prostate.

**Tuesday 13 December**

I was at The Central Clinic of Athens at 8.30 am to get hooked up to my intravenous antibiotics. The Voncon, Meronem and Zyvoxid dripped into me really quickly – much faster than previous visits.

My morning intravenous session was over by 9.45 am. I then visited the doctor to do my fourteenth uroflow test. The purpose of this was to measure my urinary efficiency ahead of this week's intraprostatic injection.

After my uroflow test I had another transrectal scan of my prostate to analyse remaining inflammation areas.

My prostate was now 33% smaller than when I started the program.

*My fourteenth uroflow test showed a much smoother urine flow, with a maximum flow of 26.9 ml/second. The doctor said this was good, but not as high as he wanted it to be.*

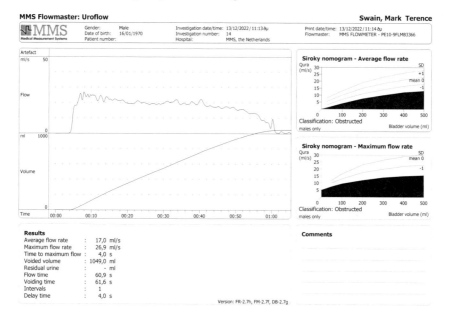

*My fifth transrectal scan showed a prostate that had reduced further in size in the last week. It now measured 10.10 ml compared to its original 15.02 ml.*

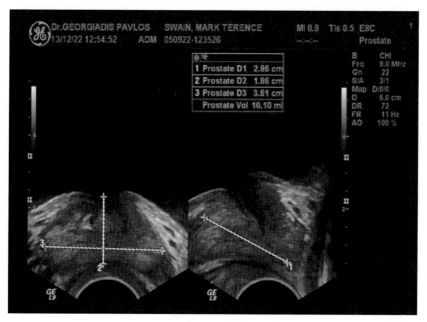

The doctor advised the majority of my remaining inflammation was where the prostate meets the urethra. It was this that was causing some slight urinary straining and restriction. Overall, the doctor was happy with the scan and advised I was 95% better now. This was the kind of news I wanted to hear.

The doctor was confident he could eliminate the remaining inflammation in this week's planned prostate injection. We followed up the transrectal scan with a prostate massage, prostate PiezoWave and penis PiezoWave.

The doctor and I then discussed how important persistence and commitment are to succeed in this program.

## There are no quick fixes to cure Chronic Prostatitis. It takes hard work from both the patient and the doctor.

At 7 pm I had my intravenous antibiotics of Voncon 250 ml, Meronem 100 ml and Zyvoxid 300 ml again. The antibiotics were over in one hour and forty-five minutes, and then I had my prostate massage and prostate PiezoWave to finish the day.

Although by now my prostate was in good shape, the doctor was still working hard on my prostate tissue that was not so soft. After my treatment, Elena, the doctor's wife, kindly offered me some desert sweets made with stevia. It was the first sweet thing I had tasted in three-and-a-half months and was absolute heaven.

I walked to the hotel glad the day of intravenous antibiotics was over.

### Wednesday 14 December

I was in The Central Clinic of Athens IV therapy ward at 8.30 am for my morning intravenous antibiotics. After one hour and forty-five minutes the Voncon, Meronem and Zyvoxid had dripped steadily into me. I noticed yesterday and today how the antibiotics seemed to be releasing and relaxing my lower stomach muscles.

After my morning antibiotics I went to the doctor for a prostate massage, prostate PiezoWave and penis PiezoWave. I was then free to eat and relax before my next batch of antibiotics.

The good news the doctor advised me today was that I would not be taking the Tygacil antibiotic as planned from tomorrow. Tygacil causes gastro sensitivity and dizziness in many patients, so I was glad to be avoiding this. The doctor said, given I was progressing well, felt fine and it seemed the microbes were not causing too many symptoms, the Tygacil could be avoided.

From 6.30 pm I took Voncon, Meronem and Zyvoxid antibiotics intravenously. It took two-and-a-half hours to finish the three bottles this time.

I then rounded the day out at the doctor's clinic having a second prostate massage and second prostate PiezoWave.

## Thursday 15 December (surgery day)

I was at The Central Clinic of Athens at 8 am for my intravenous antibiotics of Voncon, Meronem and Zyvoxid. I was certainly glad I was not having the super-strong Tygacil antibiotic as previously planned.

Each person is different in terms of the bacteria they contract and the level of resistance it has. Two people may have the same bacteria but with different resistance levels. This means different antibiotics are needed to treat it.

After my two-and-a-half hours of antibiotics I walked up to the doctor's clinic for my prostate massage, prostate PiezoWave and penis PiezoWave treatment. All my morning treatments were done by noon. I had forty-five minutes to relax in the doctor's surgery before heading back down to The Central Clinic of Athens where my surgery would take place.

*All dressed up and ready for my fourth intraprostatic injection at The Central Clinic of Athens.*

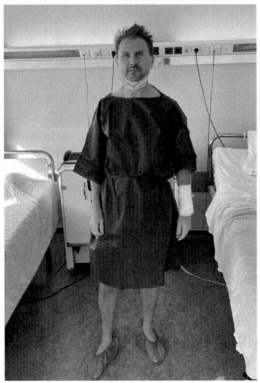

At 2.15 pm I walked with fellow patient Jacob down to the operating area.

I was soon lying on a bed and hooked up to a saline drip to provide me with some fluid and vitamins I was not able to take during the day. (No breakfast is allowed the day of the surgery.)

A friendly doctor took some blood out of my left arm to use in my PRP penis rejuvenation injection. I was then hooked up to anaesthetic in my left arm intravenous-drip-connected vein.

Soon I was in the hazy and dozy world of anaesthetic. While I was in this other world Pavlos expertly directed proceedings again and my day's menu of surgery was completed as follows:

• Urethra dilation (to widen urethra and increase urine flow).

- Fibrinolytic agent injection (to stimulate tissue repair in the penis).
- Intraprostatic injection (to target the remaining bacteria and inflammation in my lower prostate near the connection with my urethra).
- PRP penis injection (to stimulate blood flow and vessels in the penile shaft).
- PRP prostate injection (to help with increased prostate healing).

The surgery was complete after around thirty minutes. I came around in a very relaxed state, hooked up to a beeping machine monitoring my heart rate and blood pressure. I rested on a bed near the operating theatre for around twenty minutes before I was free to walk under supervision back to the IV therapy ward.

There I relaxed and rested again, continuing to fully shake off the anaesthetic. I was also able to remove the bandage that was left in my anus after the operation and clean myself up.

After a short break to grab some food, I went back to The Central Clinic of Athens at 6 pm to start my evening antibiotics. Over two hours the Voncon, Meronem and Zyvoxid dripped slowly into me. I rounded out my day of treatment with an 8.00 pm prostate PiezoWave. It was not possible to have a prostate massage after the prostate injection.

Phew! I'd done it again. I had gotten through my prostate intra-prostatic day, my fourth.

## Friday 16 December

I was back at The Central Clinic of Athens at 9.15 am for my intravenous antibiotics. The Voncon and Meronem bottles dropped smoothly into me. By the third bottle, which was Zyvoxid, the vein in my left arm was starting to feel some pain. The nurse flushed the vein out and I continued taking antibiotics again.

> One vein will not usually last the whole week of
> intravenous antibiotics. It gets tired and starts
> to block. This means a second vein needs to be
> found for the remainder of the antibiotics.

By 11 am the Zyvoxid had finished flowing and I was able to take
the short walk to the doctor's clinic. At the clinic I had the following
treatment:

- prostate PiezoWave
- penis PiezoWave.

By now I was feeling quite tired and sluggish from all the week's antibiotics. I ate some food and went to the hotel to sleep for two hours.

At 5.45 pm I was back at The Central Clinic of Athens hooked
up to antibiotics again. My vein was changed from my left arm to
my right arm after two hours of antibiotics as my left vein was really
struggling to take more. Fifteen hours of antibiotics in my left arm
had been enough, and it was starting to block and get a bit painful.
My right arm with a new vein allowed the intravenous antibiotics to
quickly drip into me again and I could quickly finish the Zyvoxid
and leave the clinic. There was now only one more set of IV antibiotics to do tomorrow morning. Yeah!

I then did a single prostate PiezoWave (due to having a sensitive
prostate after the injection yesterday, a prostate massage was not a
feasible option). By 9.30 pm I was free to go to my hotel and rest.

## Saturday 17 December

I was hooked up to antibiotics at The Central Clinic of Athens at
8 am. After two bottles, the Zyvoxid and Voncon, I took a break and
went to the doctor for my morning prostate PiezoWave and penis
PiezoWave.

At 10.30 am I then went back to the Clinic to finish my remaining bottle of antibiotics, Meronem.

I'd done it – I'd gotten through my fourth intravenous antibiotics week and my fourth intraprostatic injection. It was time to rest and relax before my last week's treatment before another two-week break. I headed off in a taxi to Zen Beach and simply sat in a deck-chair looking at the sun and sea.

## WEEK 14: Final targeting of remaining prostate inflammation before two-week antibiotic-free break from the program.

After a relaxing weekend with lots of sleep in Voula, I was back in the doctor's clinic at 11.30 on the Monday morning of week fourteen of treatment.

The doctor did a prostate massage on me (the first after my four-day break following last week's intraprostatic injection) plus my regular penis PiezoWave for sexual dysfunction and prostate PiezoWave.

I explained to him I had blood in my sperm after ejaculating last night and he said this is perfectly normal after an intraprostatic injection.

The doctor advised me this morning that when I come back in two weeks after my Christmas break, I would need to stay in Athens for a further six weeks of treatment. The doctor's plan was to carry out two further intraprostatic injections and two further penis dilations. His prognosis was that by then I would very likely be 100% cleared and free to return to normal life. His only caveat was I should continue my healthy diet for three to four months to allow the most productive prostate tissue repair.

In the early evening before my treatment, I took a walk to the main Syntagma central square in Athens to see the beautifully lit Christmas decorations. A simple and enjoyable moment like this is something I would not have done in the past.

Previously my symptoms would have made me too tired and lethargic; I'd usually say I cannot be bothered or just put things off.

I was back at the clinic in the evening at 8.15 for my second treatment of the day. I had a prostate massage to start and my prostate felt more sensitive than usual due to last week's injection. As the doctor wriggled his finger around on my prostate I was grimacing as I counted to my now familiar one hundred and fifty for each finger insertion. I had found that if I counted to one hundred and fifty in my head each massage would by then be complete. It was sometimes a long, arduous count!

There was some sensitivity and slight pain in my left flank after the massage. This was followed up with a prostate PiezoWave which was relaxing compared to the massage. The PiezoWave was over in ten minutes, and I was free to leave after checking off another day of treatment.

## Tuesday 20 December

I was at the doctor's clinic at 10.30 for my regular morning treatment of:

- Prostate massage (to break down sclerotic prostate tissue).
- Sexual dysfunction erection PiezoWave treatment (to stimulate penis blood vessels and increase erection capability).
- Prostate PiezoWave (to target central areas of infection and inflammation in my prostate).

Following my treatment, I caught up with fellow patient Thomas to interview him about his Chronic Prostatitis experience. Thomas was another poor sufferer like me, who took years to find out that he had Chronic Prostatitis.

In the evening at 7 pm I returned to the doctor's clinic for another prostate massage and prostate PiezoWave.

The doctor's focus now was to continue breaking down any long-standing hardened prostate tissue caused by years of chronic inflammation.

## Wednesday 21 December

I was back at the doctor's clinic at 10.30 am for my regular prostate massage, penis PiezoWave and prostate PiezoWave treatment.

By now I was noticing lots of fluttering and flickering taking place in my left flank and lower abdomen. It felt like real-time healing was taking place during my treatment.

The doctor and I spoke about how Chronic Prostatitis sufferers put much of their declining health and symptoms down to old age. The sufferer's brain adapts and accepts their slowly diminishing health.

This acceptance of mild symptoms and declining health takes place up to a point that the symptoms are bad enough that the brain says, 'enough, I have a problem that now needs sorting out'.

At 6 pm I had my final prostate massage and final prostate PiezoWave of the day. The flickering in my lower abdomen and left flank continued afterwards. I was convinced my body was steadily healing more.

## Thursday 22 December

This morning would be my last treatment before a two-week Christmas break from the antibiotics. From 9.30 am I completed a prostate massage and prostate PiezoWave over the next twenty minutes. I also completed my now regular penis erection PiezoWave to stimulate erectile performance.

The doctor advised when I returned to the clinic after the Christmas break, I would undergo another prostate massage followed by a sperm test to determine what bacteria (if any) were still left in my prostate. As the doctor had moved from treating the outer areas of my inflammation and infection over the last fourteen weeks towards the core of my original infection near my urethra, it would be important to find out what bacteria was left and what their levels of resistance were.

I was now free to rest and relax over the Christmas break and was advised to stop taking any antibiotics. I would be back in just over two weeks for the final push to eradicate Chronic Prostatitis and get my life back.

On the taxi ride to the airport, I was pleased to convince Mariza the taxi driver to give up smoking. I told her my prostate recovery story with all my newfound positive energy. I really was a new person heading back to Christmas in the UK, compared to the lethargic wreck I was fourteen weeks ago.

## Second break from the program. An eighteen-day Christmas break with all antibiotics stopped.

It was nice arriving home for Christmas. The first thing I noticed was how much more energy I had and how much more productive I felt.

Simple jobs like putting up the Christmas decorations and going for a walk were not a grind anymore.

My intention over this break was to fully relax, continue my healthy diet and spend quality time with friends and family. My cousin popped in to see me on Christmas Eve and was stunned at how much slimmer and healthier I looked compared to when I last played golf with him some four months ago.

It was really tricky on Christmas Day saying no to the Christmas pudding and custard as well as the homemade mince pies. I knew however that maintaining a healthy diet would ultimately see me improve faster.

One thing I did notice at my Auntie and Uncle's on Christmas Day was that I did not need to urinate.

From 11.30 am to 4.15 pm I did not need to urinate once. This was unusual for me as in the past I would have visited the toilet to urinate probably three or four times.

The only symptoms I did notice during my break were a thick yellow coating on my tongue and sometimes a very slight pain and sensitivity in my urethra at the end of my penis.

Overall though I felt like a different person compared to when I started my treatment. I was so much more productive, positive and creative. I had a dynamic outlook on life again and was looking forward to finishing my Chronic Prostatitis recovery with a final six-week push back in Athens.

## WEEK 15: Treatment starts again. Third sperm test to check for remaining bacteria. Continuation of prostate repair treatment.

### Monday 9 January

I was back in the doctor's clinic at 9.30 am on Monday. The first task was to do a transrectal scan on my prostate to see how it had progressed over the three-week break.

After my prostate scan I undertook a ten-minute prostate PiezoWave treatment to break down any remaining sclerotic hard tissue in my prostate.

I then had a prostate massage, with pressure applied across my prostate for the now familiar four sets of a fast one-hundred-and-fifty count. The prostate massage was designed to unearth any microbes in my prostate for the Mycolab sperm test that was to follow.

*My seventh transrectal prostate scan showed hardly any inflammation and a prostate that had now reduced 33.6% in size to 9.97 ml from the original 15.02 ml.*

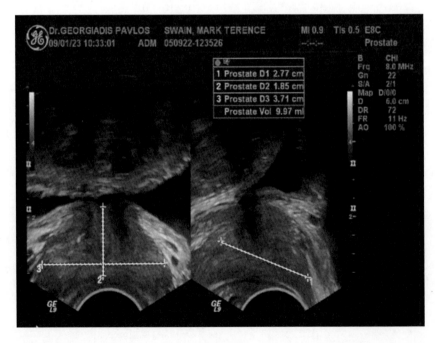

I then jumped in a taxi for the twenty-minute journey to Mycolab on the outskirts of Central Athens. There I reported to reception as before and was shown to the sterile room to deposit my sperm sample in a small plastic bottle again.

The results would be back in just over a week and would highlight if any bacteria were still present in my sperm.

The clinical specialist serving me said she hoped my microbes had gone by now. I certainly hoped so too! I was now free to go grab some lunch, rest and relax before my evening appointment at 6.30 pm.

In the evening at the doctor's, I underwent a urinary flow test to measure how my urination was performing. This was my fifteenth uroflow test. The results showed a maximum flow of 22.6 ml per second, which according to the doctor was acceptable but not at 'the gold standard' he said he wanted it to be.

*My fifteenth uroflow urine test showed the original infection was still affecting the urethra oedema. This was still causing some restriction in my urine flow.*

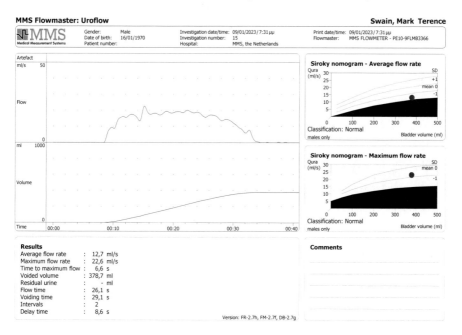

I followed up the uroflow test with a prostate PiezoWave and a hard prostate massage. After the prostate massage, for the first time my penis dripped some prostatic fluid. The fact it was watery was a good sign according to the doctor. Over the next few days, the doctor would be focusing on improving my urinary strength.

## Tuesday 10 January

I had a later appointment with the doctor today at noon. From today I was back to my regular morning daily treatment plan of:

- Prostate massage (to break down the most long-standing inflammation and sclerotic tissue in my urethra, the site of the original infection).
- Sexual dysfunction penis erection PiezoWave treatment (to stimulate penis blood vessels and further increase erection capability which was affected by the spread of microbes and inflammation).
- Prostate PiezoWave (to further target the small remaining central area of infection, inflammation and hard tissue where my prostate meets the urethra).

The prostate massage was over in about ten minutes. By now my prostate was feeling smoother and not restricted or inflamed in any way. The penis PiezoWave was performed to continue stimulating my blood vessels and the corpora cavernosa tissue, a pair of sponge-like regions of erectile tissue which contain most of the blood in the penis during an erection.

The easiest treatment was last, a painless PiezoWave sending waves up through my anus towards my prostate. As I laid on my side with the doctor holding his PiezoWave gun on my anus he was trying to break down any stubborn remaining hard tissue. The PiezoWave is also designed to promote natural healing and regeneration of healthy prostate tissue.

After lunch and some afternoon relaxation, I did my 9 pm appointment with the regular evening treatment of:

- prostate massage (to break down the limited remaining sclerotic tissue and inflammation still in my prostate at week fifteen of the program)

- prostate PiezoWave (to send electromagnetic shockwaves up through my anus towards my prostate – designed to break down any long-standing fibrotic and sclerotic tissue which had built up over years of inflammation and bacterial spread in my prostate).

The prostate massage was starting to now feel like there was not much hard or restricted area to press on. Everything inside me felt quite smooth, compared to when I started and my prostate felt hard and restricted. After four one-minute-plus cycles with the same break in between my evening prostate massage was complete. I then laid on my side for a prostate PiezoWave up through my anus towards my prostate. My second day back on treatment after the Christmas break had been ticked off.

## Wednesday 11 January

I had another noon appointment for a prostate massage, penis sexual dysfunction PiezoWave and PiezoWave on my prostate. All up this regular morning treatment took about forty-five minutes, the goal being to eliminate the final hard tissue and inflammation in my urethra.

I hadn't slept well the last two nights (and good sleep is absolutely critical during the prostate rejuvenation program). My hotel seemed to be too noisy on my return, with many loud motorbikes outside at night. The room also seemed too bright at night, and despite the staff's best efforts, the heating was too high. This combination was causing me interrupted sleep and I felt it was taking a toll on me.

It was time to move to a better, more comfortable hotel. I was happy to check in to the Heritage Hill Hotel with its ultra-comfy bed after fourteen-and-a-half weeks staying at the basic Dunlin Hotel in the rather run-down Omonia area.

I was hoping better rest and relaxation at my new hotel would aid my final recovery push.

At 8.30 pm I visited the doctor for my evening prostate massage and prostate PiezoWave. I said to the doctor my prostate actually felt tired and that it didn't want pressing any more. Maybe my tiredness was even affecting my prostate today?

I took a thirty-minute stroll back to my new hotel constantly thinking about a warm cup of tea and my comfy bed on arrival.

## Thursday 12 January

After a great night's sleep and beautiful breakfast at my new accommodation I headed to the doctor's for a 12.30 pm appointment. The regular prostate massage, penis sexual dysfunction PiezoWave and prostate PiezoWave were pretty easy to get through.

After my treatment I caught up with Hamit (whose case study you can read at the back of this book). Our discussion reminded me of what a tortuous journey many sufferers of Chronic Prostatitis go through before they are even correctly diagnosed.

At 9 pm I completed a prostate massage and prostate PiezoWave.

## Friday 13 January

I had a 1 pm appointment today and managed to get through quite a tough and strong prostate massage. To keep promoting healthy blood flow in my penis, following all the inflammation, I then had a penis PiezoWave treatment. My morning treatment was then rounded off with a prostate PiezoWave, up through my anus towards my prostate and lower urethra.

After my treatment I arranged to meet fellow patient Spiros from Brazil later in the day, whose story you can also read at the back of this book.

When I met Spiros at 7.30 pm I was surprised to hear how many of his strange symptoms were similar to mine. For instance, he had experienced really bad body aches and fibromyalgia-type symptoms. He would regularly get pain in his left thigh, bad back pain and aches all up his back.

After our meeting I had a prostate massage where the doctor pressed pretty hard on my prostate again to attack the most central part of the original long-standing fibrotic tissue. I also did a prostate PiezoWave to further help break down the hard remaining tissue.

## Saturday 14 January

My final appointment of my first week back after the Christmas break started at 9.15 am.

I had a regular prostate massage, penis PiezoWave and prostate PiezoWave treatments performed on me.

My prostate by now was a round 10 ml sponge, with a small, hardish pin-head-size piece of hard tissue in the centre. This centre was where the infection originally started years ago in my prostate, before spreading more widely. The doctor's goal was to steadily break down the outer layers to get right into the centre and eliminate all remaining hard tissue, inflammation and accompanying microbes.

By 10.15 am my first week back of treatment was complete and I was free to head off to the coast to rest and recuperate for two days.

## WEEK 16: Third sperm test results back. Further prostate massages and PiezoWave treatment to break down long-standing tissue where my urethra meets my prostate.

### Monday 16 January

Today was my birthday and I arranged a slightly later appointment with the doctor at 1 pm.

While I was in the waiting room, I met a new patient who had flown in from Romania named Doru. Doru was the same age as me and was having terrible Chronic Prostatitis symptoms in the waiting room. He was really struggling with advanced urinary urgency and was going off to pee nearly every ten minutes. It reminded me how serious the symptoms get when Chronic Prostatitis is left for a long time.

I had my regular prostate massage, penis PiezoWave and prostate PiezoWave treatment over the course of forty-five minutes.

In the afternoon I had a video chat with the doctor's son about some new technology he and a team of academics and engineers were developing to automate the prostate massage with a new intelligent probe and sensorised glove. This probe and glove would be driven by artificial intelligence and machine learning, and would allow partners or nurses to deliver accurate prostate massages on sufferers. The technology was being designed to reach Chronic Prostatitis sufferers all around the world.

In the evening at 9 pm the clinic very kindly treated me to a gluten-and-sugar-free birthday cake before my 9.30 treatment.

My birthday was rounded off with a prostate massage and prostate PiezoWave.

*Enjoying a birthday cake with fellow patients in the doctor's surgery.*
*Although the cake was sugar and gluten free it tasted really nice.*
*I felt like I was breaking my strict diet rules, but I was fine.*

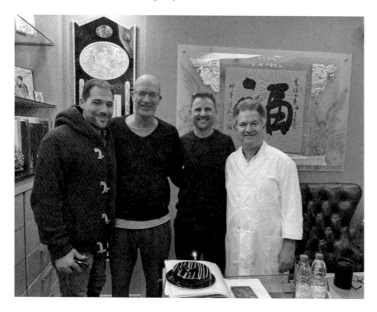

Having a prostate massage in Greece wasn't the birthday I planned last year, but I wanted to do everything I could to rid myself of this disease.

### Tuesday 17 January

While I was waiting for my 12.30 pm appointment my phone pinged with the results from my third sperm culture test.

The doctor was very pleased with these results and described them as excellent. He even said they were better than he expected, which made me very pleased. He said that I stood a very good chance of being completely clear of all microbes in my prostate within the next five weeks.

After this good news I proceeded to have my regular prostate massage, penis PiezoWave and prostate PiezoWave treatment.

*The results from my third sperm culture test showed that the klebsiella pneumoniae had been eradicated. Staphylococcus aureus was still present, but at a much lower reading of 5,000 cfu/ ml (colony forming units) compared to the original 80,000 cfu/ml.*

Ιδιωτικό Διαγνωστικό Εργαστήριο Ειδικών Λοιμώξεων - Μυκητιάσεων & Μικροβιολογικών Εξετάσεων
• Τμήμα Βιοπαθολογίας (Ορμονολογικό-Βιοχημικό-Αιματολογικό-Ανοσολογικό) - Μοριακής Βιολογίας - Προγεννητικού Ελέγχου
• Τμήμα Κυτταρολογίας - Εργαστήριο Ψηφιακής Ανάλυσης Εικόνας
(Digital Image Analysis Lab)

Λεωφ. Κηφισίας 354 Χαλάνδρι Τ.Κ. 15233
ΑΦΜ:998012799 - ΔΟΥ: ΧΑΛΑΝΔΡΙΟΥ
Τηλ. 210-8028817, 210-6890505 Φαξ: 210-6890506
www.mycolab.gr - info@mycolab.gr

Patient name:     MARK SWAIN                    DATE:     09/01/2023

## CULTURE OF SPERM

Leukocytes (White Blood Cells):   Few (10-12) per field
Stem Fungus:                      NEGATIVE (-)
Neisser:                          NEGATIVE (-)
Gramm stain:                      POSITIVE (+)

### Cultivation (aerobic)

Staphylococcus  aureus  = 5.000  cfu/ml

### Cultivation (anaerobic)

NEGATIVE (-)

### Chamydiaceae:

NEGATIVE (-)

### Mycoplasma Fermentans

NEGATIVE (-)

### Mycoplasma Hominis:

NEGATIVE (-)

### Ureaplasma Urealyticum:

NEGATIVE (-)

**COMMENTS**
PH 8.0 - Hb (+) Erythrocytes Few (6-8) per field

The Doctor

Ιδιωτικό Διαγνωστικό Εργαστήριο Ειδικών Λοιμώξεων - Μυκητιάσεων & Μικροβιολογικών Εξετάσεων
• Τμήμα Βιοπαθολογίας (Ορμονολογικό-Βιοχημικό-Αιματολογικό-Ανοσολογικό) - Μοριακής Βιολογίας - Προγεννητικού Ελέγχου
• Τμήμα Κυτταρολογίας - Εργαστήριο Ψηφιακής Ανάλυσης Εικόνας
(Digital Image Analysis Lab)

Λεωφ. Κηφισίας 354 Χαλάνδρι Τ.Κ. 15733
ΑΦΜ:998012799 - ΔΟΥ: ΧΑΛΑΝΔΡΙΟΥ
Τηλ. 210-8028817, 210-6890505 Φαξ: 210-6890506
www.mycolab.gr - info@mycolab.gr

## ANTIBIOGRAM

**MARK SWAIN**                     Athens          09/01/2023

Material :          *CULTURE OF SPERM*

Microbe :          *Staphylococcus aureus = 5.000 cfu/ml*

| | Classif/tion | MIC's | | Classif/tion | MIC's |
|---|---|---|---|---|---|
| PENICILLINE : | | | ERYTHROMYCIN: | R | |
| AMPICILLIN: | R | | CLARITHROMYCIN: | R | |
| AMOXICILLIN: | R | | ROXITHROMYCIN: | R | |
| AMOX.+AC.CLAVUL.: | S | | AZITHROMYCIN: | R | |
| AMPICIL.+SULBACT. | | | | | |
| PIPERACILLIN: | | | | | |
| PIPERACILLIN/TAZOBACTAM: | | | AZTREOENAM: | | |
| TICARCILLIN: | | | IMIPENEM: | | |
| TICARCILLIN+AC.CLAV.: | | | MEROPENEM | | |
| | | | GENTAMICIN: | S | |
| | | | TOBRAMYCIN: | | |
| CEFADROXIL: | | | NETILMYCIN: | | |
| CEPHALOTHIN: | S | | AMICACIN: | S | |
| CEPHAZOLIN: | | | TETRACYCLIN | R | |
| CEFAMANDOLE: | | | DOXYCYCLIN: | | |
| CEFOXITINE: | S | | CLINDAMYCIN: | S | |
| CEFUROXIME SODIUM: | R | | METRONIDAZOLE: | | |
| CEFUROXIME AXETIL: | R | | CHLORAMPHENICOL: | S | |
| CEFACLOR: | | | TRIMETH. SULFA: | S | |
| CEFPROZIL: | | | NITROFURANTOIN: | S | |
| CEFIXIME: | R | | ACID FUSIDIC: | S | |

1 of 2

P340e Software
210.68r2998

141

Ιδιωτικό Διαγνωστικό Εργαστήριο Ειδικών Λοιμώξεων - Μυκητιάσεων & Μικροβιολογικών Εξετάσεων
• Τμήμα Βιοπαθολογίας (Ορμονολογικό-Βιοχημικό-Αιματολογικό-Ανοσολογικό) - Μοριακής Βιολογίας - Προγεννητικού Ελέγχου
• Τμήμα Κυτταρολογίας - Εργαστήριο Ψηφιακής Ανάλυσης Εικόνας
(Digital Image Analysis Lab)

myColab

Λεωφ. Κηφισίας 354 Χαλάνδρι Τ.Κ. 15233
ΑφΜ:998012799 - ΔΟΥ: ΧΑΛΑΝΔΡΙΟΥ
Τηλ. 210-8028817, 210-6890505 Φαξ: 210-6890506
www.mycolab.gr - info@mycolab.gr

| | Classif/tion | MIC's | | Classif/tion | MIC's |
|---|---|---|---|---|---|
| CEFTRIAXONE: | | | RIFAMPICIN: | | |
| CEFOTAXIME: | | | VANCOMYCIN: | S | |
| CEFTAZIDIME: | | | TEICOPLANIN: | S | |
| CEFEPIME: | | | LINEZOLID: | S | |
| | | | NOVOBIOCIN: | S | |
| COLISTIN: | | | NORFLOXACIN: | S | |
| FOSFOMYCIN: | S | | CIPROFLOXACIN: | S | |
| MUPIROCIN: | S | | OFLOXACIN: | S | |
| TIGECYCLIN: | S | | MOXIFLOXACIN: | S | |
| | | | LEVOFLOXACIN: | S | |
| | | | NALIDIXIC ACID: | R | |

S = Sensitive        R = Resistant        MS = Moderately Resistant

Comments :   Treatment with selected light antibiotics is Recommended.
Treatment and reexamination is Recommended.
Treatment with selected light antibiotics is Recommended.
Treatment and reexamination is Recommended.

DOCTOR

2 of 2

## Wednesday 18 January

After breakfast I took my regular dose of Norocin and Augmentin antibiotics. I then headed off to my morning treatment with the doctor. I had my regular prostate massage, penis PiezoWave and prostate PiezoWave before catching up with fellow patient William.

Listening to William, I was amazed how Chronic Prostatitis can be contracted by something as simple as swimming in a contaminated swimming pool. At twenty-one years old William was the youngest patient I had met so far with the disease. It certainly showed me that Chronic Prostatitis does not discriminate by age.

In the evening I completed a prostate massage and prostate PiezoWave with the goal still to break down the small amount of inflammation I had left.

## Thursday 19 January

I had a 12.30 pm appointment for my regular triple morning treatment of:

- prostate massage
- sexual dysfunction penis erection PiezoWave treatment
- prostate PiezoWave.

After my visit to the doctor, he was straight off to The Central Clinic of Athens to perform intraprostatic injections on two patients. I therefore arranged a later 9 pm evening appointment.

I had a prostate massage where the doctor advised I still had some harder tissue to break down. This was followed by a prostate PiezoWave treatment that would further assist with the tissue breakdown.

## Friday 20 January

During my normal prostate massage, penis PiezoWave and prostate PiezoWave this morning, the doctor and I talked about how important discipline is during his Chronic Prostatitis recovery program.

Many patients struggle to avoid the cakes, sweet treats and unhealthy food that only delays their progress and ends up costing them more. Often patients also wait too long in between treatments from the doctor, which gives inflammation and infection time to grow back again.

In the evening I did another prostate massage and prostate PiezoWave, where the doctor was trying to attack the inflammation still in my urethra, causing a minor burning sensation in my penis.

## Saturday 21 January

My 9.15 am appointment comprised the usual prostate massage and PiezoWave treatments.

I mentioned to the doctor how I was now experiencing erections at night very regularly, and last night every time I woke up, I seemed to have one. The doctor said this is great progress and was a good sign.

I also explained to the doctor how I was feeling so much stronger and more creative now. I was starting to feel very optimistic about the future again and was sure that great things lay ahead. This was a stark contrast to when I arrived some five months ago where everything felt a struggle.

I also mentioned to the doctor I still had some numbness and lack of sensation in my right thigh. The doctor said this would take a few months to come back as my neural system regenerated. He also mentioned I will notice many more improvements over the coming months, as my body had steadily deteriorated with Chronic Prostatitis and those effects were slowly being unwound.

I jumped in a taxi and headed to Voula to relax by the sea for the weekend, amazed at how much more positive, dynamic and creative I was feeling.

## WEEK 17: Fifth intraprostatic injection and a full week of intravenous antibiotics.

### Monday 23 January

My first task for this week was to undertake a COVID-19 test at The Central Clinic of Athens. From tomorrow I would be back in the clinic taking intravenous antibiotics again, and I would require an all-clear showing I was free from COVID-19.

After my COVID-19 test I went to the doctor for a prostate massage, penis PiezoWave and prostate PiezoWave.

The doctor asked if I had any irritation in my penis from the urethra now and my answer was any pain was very intermittent and minor. This, according to the doctor, was a very good sign.

> The doctor also said I was now on the final rounds of the program and would soon be fully treated.

I mentioned to the doctor that today my neck and arms felt stiff and achy. I believed it was because of the Norocin and Augmentin antibiotics I was taking. The doctor agreed, but said I would be off the oral tablet antibiotics and onto intravenous ones from tomorrow.

At 9 pm I had a prostate massage and prostate PiezoWave. I asked the doctor to give his very best estimate on how long I'd had Chronic Prostatitis.

> The doctor's response was that I'd had Chronic Prostatitis for more than fifteen years and less than twenty years. This was based on the symptoms I had developed way before treatment.

## Tuesday 24 January

My day started at The Central Clinic of Athens therapy treatment room 502 at 8.30 am with fellow patient Hamit.

The friendly nurse Ellie found my vein pretty easily and the 250 ml of Voncon, 100 ml of Meronem and 300 ml of Zyvoxid dripped into me quickly over the next hour.

I found it surprising that as the antibiotics started to drip into me, my ears started to itch. I was convinced this was another weird link between the prostate and other parts of the body.

I then went to visit the doctor at his clinic just up the road. I advised him about my ears itching and he explained it may be an antifungal reaction to the intravenous antibiotics. He prescribed some Fungustatin antifungal tablets which I was to take after lunch.

I completed a prostate massage and PiezoWave treatments. The doctor advised me he would do another transrectal scan and uroflow urine test tomorrow to measure my progress. These results would be important in advance of my fifth intraprostatic injection planned for Thursday.

In the afternoon I rested and relaxed as the antibiotics were making me feel a bit weaker than normal.

In the evening I did a second round of intravenous antibiotics from 6.30 pm to 8.30 pm. The day was rounded off with a prostate massage and prostate PiezoWave.

## Wednesday 25 January

I was back in The Central Clinic of Athens at 8.30 am to start my regular morning cocktail of antibiotics. The three bottles of Voncon, Meronem and Zyvoxid were inside my body within two-and-a-half hours. I then went straight to my urologist with a full bladder to do my sixteenth uroflow test.

*My latest uroflow test showed a strong ability for my bladder to hold a large amount of urine (1304 ml) without problem. My maximum urine flow had also increased to a stronger pressure of 27.1 ml/per second.*

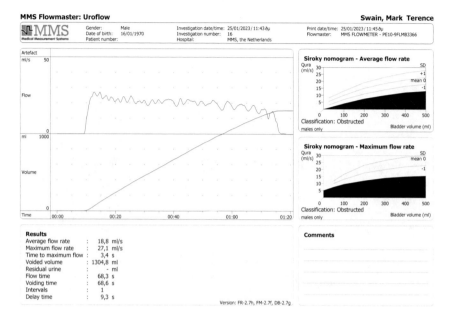

I then had another transrectal scan done to measure the inflammation still left in my prostate.

The doctor explained the latest reduction in prostate size over the last two weeks was probably due to the breaking down of an oedema.

After the scans I had my regular prostate massage, penis PiezoWave and prostate PiezoWave treatments. After an afternoon of rest, I went to Athens Clinic to undertake intravenous antibiotics from 6 till 8 pm. I then finished my day with a prostate massage and prostate PiezoWave. I then went to bed early to get plenty of rest for my intraprostatic injection day tomorrow.

*By week seventeen of treatment my prostate had very minimal inflammation. My prostate had also reduced further in size to 9.62 ml.*

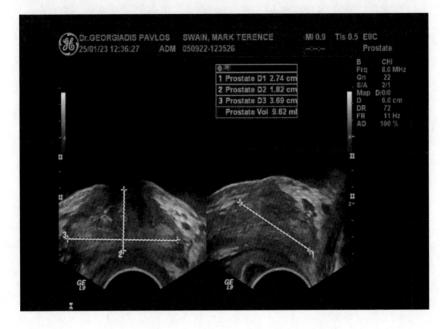

## Thursday 26 January

I had a very light breakfast due to the surgery ahead. A small tub of yogurt, slice of seeded rye bread, single kiwi fruit and glass of water was my start to the day.

My menu of treatment planned for today was:

- PRP prostate injection (to regenerate and rejuvenate healthy tissue in my prostate affected by long-standing inflammation).
- PRP penis injection (to regenerate and rejuvenate healthy tissue in my penis affected by long-standing inflammation).
- Intraprostatic injection (an injection of antibiotics into my prostate to help kill the remaining staphylococcus aureus bacteria present).
- Fibrinolytic agent (an injection of a special agent to help disintegrate hard tissue that had built up in my penis and prostate).

- Urethral dilatation (a widening of the urethra to help urine flow given inflammation over the years had caused urinary restriction).

My first task was to head to The Central Clinic of Athens for intravenous antibiotics. I took 250 ml of Voncon, 100 ml of Meronem and 300 ml of Zyvoxid between 9 and 11.30 am. It was then a short walk to the doctor's for a prostate massage, penis PiezoWave and prostate PiezoWave.

With little time to rest, I had to go back to The Central Clinic of Athens to get ready for surgery.

*Dressed and ready for my fifth intraprostatic injection.*

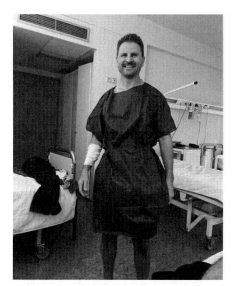

I was soon asked to walk down to the operating area of the clinic with a senior nurse, who asked me to lay on a bed and covered me with a blanket. The assistant surgeon then drew three vials of blood from my left arm. Following this I was taken to the main operating theatre where liquid anaesthetic was injected into my right arm and an oxygen mask applied on my face.

Before I knew it, I was in the hazy and dozy world of anaesthesia once again and slowly drifted off. I was awoken abruptly by a nurse to advise the operation was over. I was wheeled back to the intravenous antibiotics therapy ward to recuperate and shake off the anaesthetics.

The bottle of water I was given felt great after seven hours without drinking. Intraprostatic injection five was over and I could lay on my hospital bed to get back to full alertness. After feeling ready to leave the clinic, I grabbed a quick bite to eat with fellow patient Hamit. We then returned to finish our evening intravenous antibiotics between 6 and 8.30 pm.

The huge day was rounded off with a prostate PiezoWave only.

## Friday 27 January

It took four hours for my antibiotics to drip into me this morning as my right arm vein was accepting the fluids very slowly.

After changing the cannula to my left arm things started to speed up. By 1.45 pm the three bottles of antibiotics were inside me. I grabbed a quick vegetable and wholegrain pasta lunch bowl at Cultivos cafe before heading to the doctor's surgery for my treatment of a penis PiezoWave and prostate PiezoWave.

After some rest in the afternoon, I was back at The Central Clinic of Athens for intravenous antibiotics between 6.45 and 8.45 pm. I then headed to the doctor's waiting room where I struck up a conversation with new patient John. Our discussion highlighted to me how Chronic Prostatitis can cause major depression in sufferers.

My evening treatment with the doctor comprised only a prostate PiezoWave. I now had only one more set of intravenous antibiotics to do tomorrow morning before the week's treatment was over.

## Saturday 28 January

I had my intravenous antibiotics from 8.45 am to 10.45 am. It was then time to visit the doctor for a penis PiezoWave and prostate

PiezoWave treatment. The doctor explained to me that many patients struggle with sticking to the prescribed diet during treatment. One of his patients was still eating white bread, despite it being high in carbohydrates and a favourite food of the staphylococcus microbe.

> I will reinforce it again: it is critical to have the discipline to stick to your prescribed diet to recover from Chronic Prostatitis.

## WEEK 18: Back to daily prostate massages to break down any final remaining hard prostate tissue.

### Monday 30 January

The goal this week was to break down any remaining hard tissue in my prostate that may still be home for the staphylococcus aureus bacteria.

I did a prostate massage, penis PiezoWave and prostate PiezoWave treatment at 11 am. The doctor said my prostate was now in very good shape and felt smooth, with only some minor hard tissue areas.

We spoke about how my mother's neighbour had developed prostate cancer and had some of his prostate removed.

> The sufferer's wife said he had lost his 'male libido' and 'felt like a woman' due to part of his prostate being removed.

The doctor explained to me that his prostate cancer was almost certainly caused by bacterial Chronic Prostatitis being left untreated for many years. This comment made me even more thankful I was getting treatment for the disease.

I rested in the afternoon as I was still somewhat tired from last week's very strong intravenous antibiotic load.

Before my appointment in the evening I caught up with fellow patient Paul. Our discussion reminded me of how serious the urinary symptoms can be with Chronic Prostatitis.

I then visited the doctor to finish the day with a prostate massage and prostate PiezoWave. I mentioned to the doctor I was now experiencing a flickering sensation regularly in my left flank. His response was my neural nerve endings were recovering and this muscular fibrillation was a sign of healing.

## Tuesday 31 January

I had a later 1 pm appointment today. While in the waiting room, I started chatting to new patient George, from Crete.

It was very interesting to hear how thirty-five-year-old George also experienced severe lethargy and tiredness during his worst Chronic Prostatitis symptoms, like I did. After our discussion I visited the doctor's treatment room for my regular prostate massage, penis PiezoWave and prostate PiezoWave treatment.

After an afternoon rest, I finished the day with another prostate massage and prostate PiezoWave to break down any hardened prostate tissue remaining.

## Wednesday 1 February

At 1 pm I had an uneventful prostate massage, penis PiezoWave and prostate PiezoWave.

In the evening at 8 pm I had a prostate massage and prostate PiezoWave. I was by now feeling pretty much no pain while having the prostate massage. The only point of mild sensitivity was near my urethra. Overall, now the pain I previously experienced during a prostate massage had largely disappeared.

## Thursday 2 February

I had a prostate massage, penis erection PiezoWave and prostate massage at 11.30 am.

Following my treatment, I had lunch with George. It was really interesting to hear how when George was stressed and he led a less healthy lifestyle – consuming alcohol and smoking – his symptoms were much, much worse.

After doing some work in the afternoon (I had much more energy now), I visited the doctor in the evening for a prostate massage and prostate PiezoWave.

## Friday 3 February

I had a 12.30 pm appointment with the doctor. I completed a prostate massage, penis erection PiezoWave and prostate PiezoWave as normal.

The doctor and I talked about how close I was to eradicating all microbes and finishing the treatment. The doctor said it was difficult to tell until my next transrectal scan exactly how long this would take. He said I should expect to possibly have to extend my stay for a further few weeks. Everything would be dependent on my next scan, planned for 14 February before my next intraprostatic injection.

In the evening at 9.30 pm I did a prostate massage and prostate PiezoWave. I was amazed at the energy I had afterwards while walking to the metro station. I was able to run up the flights of stairs with seemingly boundless energy.

I seemed to have the energy I had twenty-five years ago and was feeling incredible.

## Saturday 4 February

At 9.30 am I had my regular morning prostate massage, penis erection PiezoWave and prostate PiezoWave to round off the week's treatment. The PiezoWave generated some sharp shooting nerve feelings in my penis, which I hoped was due to further hard prostate tissue near the urethra breaking down.

After my appointment I stocked up on Norocin and Augmentin antibiotic tablets. I continued to take these tablets after breakfast and my evening meal every day. These tablets alongside my physical treatment were designed to help eliminate the remaining bacteria in my prostate.

## WEEK 19: Continued oral antibiotics and daily physical therapy to target the few remaining staphylococcus aureus bacteria.

### Monday 6 February

I was surprised to wake up to see snow falling in the Athens area. I made my way in the three degrees Celsius temperatures to my 12.30 pm appointment. At the clinic I had a prostate massage, penis PiezoWave and prostate PiezoWave over the next forty-five minutes.

The doctor said I should work hard to avoid consuming any pepper and spicy food in my diet. He mentioned I should in particular look out for foods that have pepper added before they are cooked as this could act as an irritant for the prostate inflammation.

Overall, in the doctor's opinion my prostate was soft and I was getting closer to the end of the program. I certainly hoped so!

After a rest in the afternoon, I travelled to the doctor's clinic for my 9 pm appointment. While waiting for my appointment I discussed the importance of prostate injections with fellow patients Hamit and Panos. Both of them felt that intraprostatic injections are crucial for a recovery from Chronic Prostatitis. Panos, who had just had his first prostate injection, mentioned that his prostatitis symptoms and prostate were noticeably better after his first injection.

Following our discussion, I was called to the doctor's treatment room to undertake my prostate massage and prostate PiezoWave.

## Tuesday 7 February

I had a 1 pm appointment today to massage my prostate and have piezo shockwaves sent through my perineum towards my prostate. The doctor was still trying to break down any hard tissue on my prostate that may still contain bacteria.

I also had a penis erection PiezoWave treatment to stimulate blood vessels and assist with erectile performance.

After my treatment, I caught up with fellow patient Dimos, who had just undergone his first prostate PiezoWave treatment. He mentioned, like me, how he noticed a connection between the prostate and ear during the treatment. He summarised this connection well:

> 'The prostate PiezoWave seemed to unclear my ear that had felt partly blocked for a long time.'

In the evening at 9 pm, I also did a prostate massage and prostate PiezoWave.

## Wednesday 8 February

Today, I did a slightly later 2 pm prostate massage, penis erection PiezoWave and prostate PiezoWave.

In the evening before my appointment, I spoke to fellow patient Vassilis, who had been suffering from Chronic Prostatitis for over twenty years.

I was then called into the doctor's surgery to have a prostate massage and prostate PiezoWave to round out the day.

## Thursday 9 February

Before my morning appointment I spoke to the doctor's wife Elena about the importance of a positive mental attitude while going through the Chronic Prostatitis treatment program.

Elena mentioned to me how she had generally seen positive patients progress much more quickly through the program and heal faster. After our chat I had my normal prostate massage, penis erection PiezoWave and prostate PiezoWave treatment in a positive frame of mind.

In the evening I did a 9 pm prostate massage and prostate PiezoWave.

## Friday 10 February

My first appointment was at 12.30 pm and the doctor focused his attention during my prostate massage on breaking down and smoothing out any harder sclerotic prostate tissue. He advised these are the areas inflammation and bacteria could still be hiding. He also said I was right near the end of the treatment program, which I found reassuring.

Following my thorough prostate massage, I did a penis erection PiezoWave and prostate PiezoWave.

Early in the evening I met fellow patient Vassilis (whose story you can read at the back of this book). I was astounded to hear Chronic Prostatitis caused Vassilis so much pain that he struggled to get out of bed for twenty days. Vassilis, like myself, felt delighted when he was finally diagnosed accurately with Chronic Prostatitis. It allowed him to stop worrying, which was likely making his symptoms worse.

Following our discussion, I rounded out the day with a prostate massage and prostate PiezoWave.

## Saturday 11 January

To finish off my week of treatment I had my usual combination of a prostate massage, penis PiezoWave and prostate PiezoWave. The doctor said each of these three treatments was working in their own distinct way to rejuvenate my entire urogenital system. The prostate massage was smoothing out the hard sclerotic tissue on my prostate, the penis PiezoWave was stimulating the cavernous tissue in my penis and the prostate PiezoWave was breaking down any final-long standing fibrotic tissue on my prostate.

# WEEK 20: Sixth intraprostatic injection and full week of intravenous antibiotics.

## Monday 13 February

I started my twentieth week of treatment with a prostate massage. The doctor focused heavily on the point my urethra connected to my prostate. This was the point of my original infection and the doctor had 'broken down the outer layers' to now attack this core area.

Following the prostate massage, I did a penis erection PiezoWave and prostate PiezoWave.

In the evening before my appointment, I chatted with fellow patient Doru from Romania. Like me, he had excruciating back pain as one of his Chronic Prostatitis symptoms. Unlike me, he did not just visit one urologist, he visited over a dozen. In fact, he had been searching in his home country for over ten years for a cure to his problems.

At 9 pm I went into the doctor's treatment room for a prostate massage and prostate PiezoWave. I then went to bed early to get some sleep before my intravenous antibiotics would start tomorrow.

## Tuesday 14 February

I arrived at The Central Clinic of Athens at 9.40 am to start my intravenous antibiotics. These antibiotics would help prepare me for my sixth prostate injection this coming Thursday and help fight any bacteria left in my prostate.

It took one hour forty-five minutes for the Voncon, Zyvoxid and Meronem to drip steadily into me.

After my antibiotics I took the short walk to the doctor's clinic for my morning treatment. The first thing I did was a uroflow test to measure how efficient my urination was. I could sense the doctor was not happy with the result.

My maximum flow rate of 22.4 ml/per second was worse than prior tests. This showed the staphylococcus aureus was still causing a restriction in my urethra.

157

Following the uroflow test I had my eighth transrectal ultra-sound. This scan supported my lower urinary flow measurement.

*My seventeenth uroflow test showed a maximum flow rate of 22.4 ml/second.*

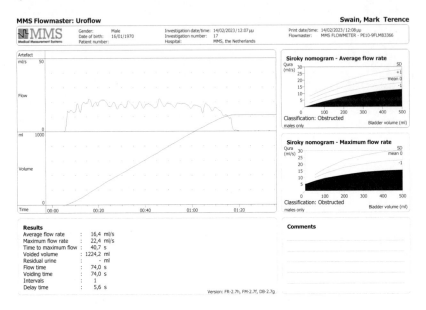

*My eighth prostate transrectal scan still showed some inflammation caused by microbes in my urethra.*

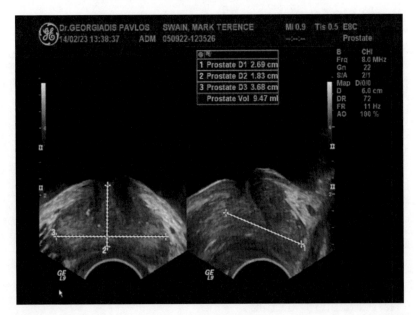

The inflammation in my urethra demonstrated bacteria were still present. The doctor said this was the point of the original infection many years ago and I now needed to cut back on any carbohydrates, including dark bread, wholegrain pasta, rice and potatoes. The staphylococcus aureus was still surviving on what little carbohydrates I was eating.

I felt a bit down today having a transrectal scan that still showed inflammation and a materially worse urinary performance. I vowed from today I would starve the staphylococcus and not eat a single carbohydrate until they were eradicated.

After my scan I had my regular morning routine of a prostate massage, penis erection PiezoWave and prostate PiezoWave. After a short break from 4 to 7 pm, I went back to The Central Clinic of Athens for my second batch of antibiotics for the day. Between 7 and 9.30 pm all three bottles of antibiotics slowly dripped into me. Following this I visited the doctor for a prostate massage and prostate PiezoWave.

The doctor and I then spoke about the best foods to eat to minimise my carbohydrate intake. The keto-style diet was recommended to me, which would be the best approach to stop feeding the staphylococcus aureus bacteria, which are notoriously difficult to eliminate.

## Wednesday 15 February

I was back at The Central Clinic of Athens at 9.40 am for my three bottles of antibiotics; Voncon, Zetalid and Meronem.

The intravenous antibiotics dripped into me over a period of five-and-a-half hours. Today my vein seemed to be much slower accepting the fluids, especially the second bottle which was the stronger Zetalid, which dripped into me at a snail's pace.

After this I visited the doctor's clinic for a prostate massage, penis PiezoWave and prostate PiezoWave. I had a brief three-hour rest before heading back to the doctor's clinic for another prostate massage and prostate PiezoWave.

At 9.30 pm I went to The Central Clinic of Athens for two more hours of intravenous antibiotics. While I was there, I chatted to fellow patient Nikos, who even had swollen feet as a symptom of Chronic Prostatitis.

## Thursday 16 February

I was back at the doctor's clinic at 9.30 am for a prostate massage, penis erection PiezoWave and prostate PiezoWave. I was feeling tired today due to a mix of the intravenous antibiotics and the fact I was cutting back on carbohydrates.

At 10.30 am I started my intravenous antibiotics for the day, which were much faster, dripping into me over the next two-and-a-half hours.

Before I knew it, I was asked to change into my surgery gown and plastic socks again. I was soon back in the operating theatre having blood withdrawn from my left arm for use in the PRP injection in my penis and prostate. The PRP injection is designed to stimulate and rejuvenate any damaged areas. My full menu of surgery today would be:

- Urethra dilation (to widen my urethra and increase urine flow).
- Fibrinolytic agent injection (to stimulate tissue repair in the penis).
- Intraprostatic injection (to target the remaining bacteria and inflammation in my lower prostate near the connection with my urethra).
- PRP penis injection (to stimulate blood flow and vessels in the penile shaft).
- PRP prostate injection (to help with increased prostate healing).

At 3 pm, I awoke out of my anaesthetic daze and was wheeled on a hospital trolley back to the intravenous antibiotic therapy room to rest and recuperate.

The lamb and vegetables meal after the surgery tasted delicious as I was absolutely starving, due to eating no breakfast before the surgery. I rested for three hours before heading to the doctor for only a prostate PiezoWave. Following this I completed my huge day with antibiotics between 9.30 pm and midnight.

## Friday 17 February

I was back in The Central Clinic of Athens at 10 am to continue my intravenous antibiotics. All three bottles were finished by 12.15 pm. Following this I walked up to the doctor's clinic for a penis PiezoWave and prostate PiezoWave. A prostate massage was not permitted after yesterday's injection.

I had a longer break this afternoon to rest and relax before recommencing my second batch of antibiotics in the evening between 8 and 9.45 pm, which were:

- Voncon 250 ml
- Meronem 100 ml
- Zyvoxid 300 ml

I then went for a quick prostate PiezoWave before heading home to rest.

It was amazing tonight how I was absolutely craving a pain aux raisin French pastry. It was as if the microbes were finally dying and clinging to life, asking for food.

The doctor explained how the microbes will send signals to the brain to get you to feed them with sweets or carbohydrates.

161

### Saturday 18 February

I woke up without any cravings for sweet pastries and headed to the doctor's clinic for my 10 am appointment. I had a penis erection PiezoWave and prostate PiezoWave done over the next twenty-five minutes.

From there it was back to The Central Clinic of Athens for three-and-a-half hours of intravenous antibiotics between 11 am and 2.30 pm. I had a rest and relaxed in the afternoon before heading back to the doctor at 7.30 pm for a prostate PiezoWave. I completed my week of antibiotics with an intravenous session between 8.30 and 10.15 pm.

I'd done it. I'd made it through the twentieth week of treatment and my sixth intraprostatic injection.

## WEEK 21: Post-injection monitoring and prostate massage recommencement.

### Monday 20 February

I was back at the doctor to start week twenty-one of my prostate rejuvenation program at 12.30 pm.

The doctor completed a prostate massage on me again (my first since last week's injection). My urethra and prostate felt smoother and less blocked.

This was followed by a penis erection PiezoWave and prostate PiezoWave. During the prostate PiezoWave, I felt a tingling sensation in the end of my penis. The doctor advised this was due to still having some blocked nerves caused by my prostate.

I discussed with the doctor how much longer my treatment would take. He said I would need to do another prostate injection in three weeks. He said he did not want me leaving Greece until I was finally cured.

After an afternoon of rest I went back to the doctor for my second visit of the day at 9 pm.

En route to the doctor's clinic I stopped in at my regular pharmacy to weigh myself.

*I was surprised to be weighing in at 70 kg with my clothes on. Cutting down carbohydrates and sugars was reducing my weight fast from my original 78.5 kg at the start of the program.*

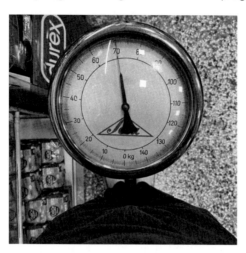

My day was rounded off with a prostate massage and prostate PiezoWave.

## Tuesday 21 February

I had my first appointment today at 12.30 pm. It was my usual prostate massage, penis erection PiezoWave and prostate PiezoWave.

The doctor's wife gave me some super bread with seeds and strong rye content, given I was low on energy today with my recent cut back on carbohydrates.

I relaxed in the afternoon as I felt pretty tired after the morning's treatment. In the evening at 8.30 pm I had a prostate massage and prostate PiezoWave. Before my evening appointment I was talking to fellow patient Nikos and the doctor's wife Elena. Nikos and I were talking about our original symptoms of Chronic Prostatitis which made me look back on my prior medical records.

*My medical records were clearly indicating all the symptoms of Chronic Prostatitis. Unfortunately, no Australian doctor or urologist was able to diagnose me with the condition.*

Thank you for seeing Mr Mark Terence Swain for opinion and management of left lower back pain associated with left flank and testicular pain. Mark has seen a number of doctors since this began in December 2019.
Character - dull ache, always there but fluctuates, doesnt affect sleep. Bending forward can aggravate.
Seen here in Dec/Jan, thoroughly investigated, no signs infection, CT abdo/pelvis NAD, testicular u/s NAD
Had u/s for hernia with GP in manly - NAD
Saw gastroenterologist Manly - NAD. recommend review with rheumatologist
I considered a radiculopathy so ordered MRI lumbar spine which showed mild L5/S1 disc protrusion however I don't think this would explain his symptoms. His lower limb neuro exam was largely unremarkable aside from slight reduced power in L5/S1 myotome on left (still 5/5).
He has recently seen rheumatologist Dr Les Schrieber who thought msk/radiculopathy was unlikely and that we should explore a urological cause.

**Medical History:**
11/10/2019 Dysuria
21/11/2019 Mastoiditis
20/01/2020 UTI

**Current Medication:**
Salbutamol CFC-Free 100mcg/dose Inhaler    1-2 puffs prn

**Allergies:**

Nil known

Kind Regards,

Before leaving the clinic for the evening I spoke to fellow patient Panegotis. He explained to me how he originally had seventeen symptoms of Chronic Prostatitis before starting his treatment.

## Wednesday 22 February

I had my prostate massage, penis erection PiezoWave and prostate PiezoWave at 2 pm today.

I explained to the doctor how I was getting erections whenever resting for a siesta or at night. His response, as usual, was, 'Bravo! Everything is going well.' The doctor explained to me I had a maximum of six weeks of treatment left before I would be free to leave Greece totally cured.

In the evening I did a prostate massage and prostate PiezoWave to continue breaking down any long-standing inflammation in my urethra.

## Thursday 23 February

I had an earlier appointment with the doctor today at 10.30 am as he was busy doing intraprostatic injections on other patients later. My regular prostate massage, penis PiezoWave and prostate PiezoWave were over in forty-five minutes.

I was free to have a longer afternoon rest than normal.

In the evening at 9.30 I did a prostate massage and prostate PiezoWave. It seemed tonight I wanted to urinate quite a lot for some reason. I went to the toilet twice at the doctor's surgery and once as soon as I got home. So, a total of three pees in one-and-a-half hours.

This worried me a little and I planned to discuss this with the doctor the next day.

## Friday 24 February

My appointment was at 2 pm today due to the doctor being very busy. I had a very firm prostate massage. It seemed by now I could take absolutely any pressure applied to my prostate and urethra by the doctor.

This was followed up with a penis erection PiezoWave to stimulate the blood vessels in my penis. I then had a prostate PiezoWave.

I talked to fellow patients Doru and George about how much commitment was needed for the program while I awaited my evening appointment. At 9 pm I had a prostate massage and a prostate PiezoWave.

Many fellow patients kept saying to me that they thought I was finishing the program now. I explained I had a few more weeks left to go.

### Saturday 25 February

I had a 10 am appointment before my long public holiday weekend break. Monday would be a day off from treatment due to a national Greek day off for Clean Monday.

I had my usual prostate massage, penis erection PiezoWave and prostate PiezoWave. The doctor said he was still pressing hard on my prostate to eliminate any sclerotic tissue where microbes may be hiding out.

> After forty-five minutes of treatment, I was free to go and relax for a long weekend. Yay!

## WEEK 22: Further prostate massages and prostate symptom monitoring.

### Tuesday 28 February

I was back at the doctor's clinic at 1 pm, following my long weekend with no treatment.

It was not pleasant going back to the clinic to be lubricated up with the doctor's finger inside me for another prostate massage, particularly given that the doctor seemed to be pressing on my prostate harder than normal this morning and twirling his finger around while pressing near my urethra!

I then did a penis erection PiezoWave where the shockwaves were triggered into my erect penis to continue stimulating cavernous tissue and blood flow. Following this it was a pretty simple prostate PiezoWave through which I nearly nodded off. From 2.30 pm I could relax until my evening appointment, which entailed another prostate massage and prostate PiezoWave.

## Wednesday 1 March

The first thing I had to do this morning was visit the Aliens Bureau in Tavros, Athens, which is essentially the police department that handles visa extensions.

My Australian visa only entitled me to stay in Greece for a maximum of ninety days during a period of one hundred and eighty days. My time limit would be expiring in a couple of weeks so I needed a visa extension to continue my medical treatment (which was not too difficult to obtain once I had the documentation in order).

Many people embarking on this treatment program may face the same situation, and the fine for overstaying your visa in Greece can be in excess of one thousand euros.

After this I visited the doctor for a 1.30 pm prostate massage, penis PiezoWave and prostate PiezoWave. In the evening I did another prostate massage and prostate PiezoWave; the prostate massage was challenging as usual.

## Thursday 2 March

With the Greece metro train strike taking place today I had a later first appointment at 2 pm. It was my usual prostate massage, penis erection PiezoWave and prostate PiezoWave.

The doctor said to me the plan would be to have two more intra-prostatic injections over the next five weeks before I would be free to leave Greece.

In the evening at 9.30 I did a prostate massage and prostate PiezoWave.

## Friday 3 March

I did a noon prostate massage, penis erection PiezoWave and prostate PiezoWave.

As the doctor twirled his finger on my prostate near my urethra, I felt pains in the end of my penis. The doctor said it was probably left over microbes and inflammation.

I discussed the remainder of my treatment plan with the doctor; to be honest, I was starting to get frustrated with how long the program was starting to drag on for and the fact it seemed to keep extending.

I knew there was no quick fix for Chronic Prostatitis, however I never expected things to take as long as they had. Also, I did not expect the day in, day out grind to be as difficult as it was.

At 9 pm I did a prostate massage and prostate PiezoWave. I also had a chat with a previous patient Stoian in America who had undergone an intensive treatment program like myself. Stoian explained to me how he undertook a total of twenty prostate injections. I hoped, and indeed prayed, I would not need as many. I was about to have my seventh.

## Saturday 4 March

The doctor explained to me that his sole focus over the weeks ahead was attacking where my urethra met my prostate. He explained in simple terms that this was the microbes' original castle and site of the original infection. The doctor's last injection had blown up the castle but he needed to ensure there were no shelters bacteria were still hiding in.

Because this is the most difficult place for the doctor to access, the two upcoming intraprostatic injections would be crucial.

I finished the week with my usual prostate massage with a focus near the urethra. I also did a penis PiezoWave and prostate PiezoWave.

I was now free to go and recharge my batteries before next week's intraprostatic injection, my seventh.

## WEEK 23: Intraprostatic injection seven. The goal being to kill any minor remaining prostate microbes once and for all.

### Monday 6 March

After a nice weekend break it was back to reality at the doctor's Asklipiou Street, Central Athens Clinic at 1 pm.

> By now I was feeling like I hardly had any symptoms at all. Maybe occasionally I had some very mild penile burning.

My first task was to go and get a COVID-19 test at The Central Clinic of Athens to confirm I would be all clear to start my intravenous antibiotics tomorrow.

I then did a prostate massage through which my prostate felt stronger, possibly from the weekend break. I also did the penis erection PiezoWave and prostate PiezoWave. I then took lunch with fellow patient Dimos before relaxing late in the afternoon.

In the evening at 9.30 I did another prostate massage and prostate PiezoWave. I also talked to the doctor about how some patients were not sticking to the dietary requirements of the program and were obviously experiencing more extreme symptoms than necessary.

### Tuesday 7 March

I was in The Central Clinic of Athens intravenous therapy ward at 10 am to start my intravenous antibiotics for the week. Over two-and-a-half hours the antibiotics slowly dripped into me. Intravenous intraprostatic injection week seven had started.

I then went to the doctor for a pre-surgery assessment of my urination and prostate.

*My nineteenth uroflow test was my first one with a maximum flow over 30 ml per second. I was very happy with my 30.6 ml per second maximum speed, which was noticeably better than my last uroflow test.*

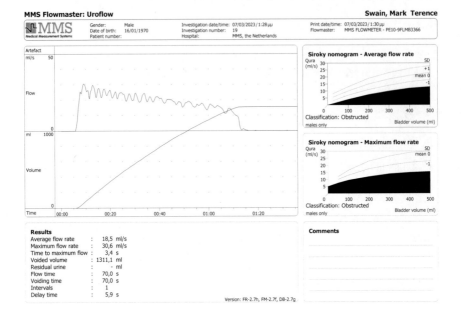

Following the uroflow test I had a transrectal image scan done to check the status of my prostate.

## My prostate was now over 40% smaller than when I started the program.

The doctor said I still had one remaining spot of inflammation where my prostate met the lower penile urethra. The doctor's plan was to blast the bacteria in this area with a bazooka cocktail of very strong antibiotics in two days.

Following the examinations, I had my normal prostate massage (not painful) and a penis erection PiezoWave and prostate PiezoWave.

I was happy to leave the doctor's clinic and felt very positive with my latest results. It was nice to rest for a few hours in the afternoon knowing such progress had taken place.

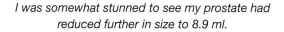

*I was somewhat stunned to see my prostate had reduced further in size to 8.9 ml.*

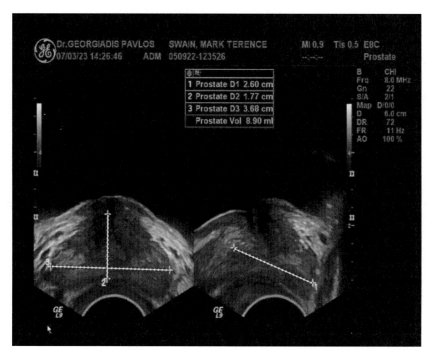

At 8 pm I was back on the intravenous antibiotics for the next two-and-a-quarter hours. This was followed by a prostate massage and prostate PiezoWave to end the day.

## Wednesday 8 March

Again, I was hooked up to my intravenous antibiotics at 10 am. The four bottles dripped into me over the next two-and-a-half hours. I then walked the five minutes to the doctor's clinic and did a prostate massage, penis PiezoWave and prostate PiezoWave.

With protests on the streets of Athens due to a recent deadly train crash on the government-run system, I took a taxi back to my hotel to rest in the afternoon and avoid the brewing trouble.

In the evening I did a further two hours of intravenous antibiotics followed by a prostate massage and prostate PiezoWave.

> The intravenous antibiotics are taken the same week as the intraprostatic injection in the prostate to provide the maximum attack against the harmful bacteria hiding out in the prostate.

### Thursday 9 March

Today was the day of my seventh intraprostatic injection. I started the day at 11 am with a very hard prostate massage in advance of the surgery. The doctor wanted to disturb all the bacteria he could that was hiding out in any fibrotic tissue. This would also give the antibiotics in the prostate injection mixture maximum impact.

I followed this up with a penis erection PiezoWave and prostate PiezoWave. I was then straight down to The Central Clinic of Athens for intravenous antibiotics between noon and 2 pm.

The prostate injection surgery was planned for 2 pm but due to delays in the operating theatre because of an earlier complex operation, the injection actually took place at 4.30 pm.

For the injection, I was basically wheeled into the operating theatre on a hospital trolley. I was then moved onto an operating table where I underwent a strong anaesthetic to knock me out so surgery could commence. Twenty minutes later, I was wheeled back out in a groggy state and was left to recoup for twenty minutes in the recovery ward. After a further hour of rest, I was free to leave the clinic.

After one hour I took the bandage out that was lodged in my backside, knowing the following procedure was over.

This is what had been done:

- Urethra dilation (to widen urethra and increase urine flow).
- Fibrinolytic agent injection (to stimulate tissue repair in the penis).
- Intraprostatic injection (to target the remaining bacteria and inflammation in my lower prostate near the connection with my urethra).
- PRP penis injection (to stimulate blood flow and vessels in the penile shaft).
- PRP prostate injection (to help with increased prostate healing).

I joined fellow patient George, who also underwent surgery, and his friend Johan for a nice grilled salmon and boiled vegetables meal after the surgery. It was then a quick walk up to the doctor's clinic for a post-surgery prostate PiezoWave.

The day's final antibiotics dripped into me between 10 pm and midnight. I noticed that the antibiotics seemed to make breathing a little more difficult and generated some tightness in my chest. However, my huge prostate injection day was over once again and I was thankfully free to head to my comfortable hotel bed.

## Friday 10 March

I was in The Central Clinic of Athens at 10 am to start intravenous antibiotics again. After two-and-a-half hours all of them had dripped into me. I then walked up to the doctor's clinic to wait for my appointment.

I urinated while waiting for the doctor and noticed the flow was much stronger and needed no straining.

The doctor performed a penis erection PiezoWave on my erect penis which did not feel so strained and painful when erect. He said it was because the injection yesterday had released urethra pressure which made my penile urethra more flexible and free.

I then did a prostate PiezoWave through which I nearly fell asleep. My morning treatment was complete. After some lunch and a siesta in the afternoon I awoke to get ready for my evening appointment.

> I felt as if a wave of happiness hit me as I walked to my evening appointment. I was singing and walking with a bounce in my step.

This super-happy feeling had happened to me three or four times throughout the program. It was as if when the microbes were being killed off in large numbers (as they would have been yesterday) I became happier.

The doctor had previously told me that the microbes were responsible for 'brain fog' and triggering me to crave sugars and carbohydrates that feed them. Obviously, my injection yesterday had killed off a large number of microbes near my urethra. Was this the reason for my elevated happiness?

It almost felt like an out-of-body experience, but coming up from inside my body. There was nothing else in particular that happened that would make me feel so happy. I hadn't won a new contract at work, spoken to a family member or received any particularly good news.

> It was just a feeling of happiness that welled up from deep inside me.

This feeling made me even more convinced there was some kind of link between killing off the microbes and my general happiness.

I was also feeling by now that my brain looked forward to taking in new information at the start of each day and learning new things. This was different from the recent past when I woke up unable to clearly think and felt lethargic.

Before my treatment started, I would usually wake up lacking energy and focus in the morning and my thinking never seemed sharp or clear. I had also spoken to many other patients who had experienced these same 'brain fog' symptoms from Chronic Prostatitis.

In the evening I was back on intravenous antibiotics at 8 pm. The antibiotics dripped into a new vein very fast over one-and-a-half hours. It was then to the doctor at 9.45 pm for a prostate PiezoWave to round out the day.

## Saturday 11 March

I visited the doctor before my intravenous antibiotics today. Given my prostate could still not be massaged following Thursday's injection, my treatment started with a penis erection PiezoWave.

The erection was much less of a strain for me today due to Thursday's injection that released my urethra. I was really starting to closely observe how every part of my body was interlinked to other parts, particularly as it related to my urogenital system.

It was amazing to me for instance how my urine flow was so much more free, easy and less strained since my last injection. It was becoming more obvious to me that I had been straining while urinating for many years. This had also caused some of the pain in the left flank of my body over a long time.

After discussing my wave of happiness that I experienced yesterday with the doctor and the potential link to the microbes, I was off for some more intravenous antibiotics.

The doctor said to me before leaving that according to recent scientific research there is a theory that the microbes almost have a thinking power.

The microbes have an ability to make you feel melancholic and unmotivated. They also have an amazing ability to make you crave the bad foods that they want to eat. I made a note to very closely observe my body's reactions over the coming weeks and months.

My intravenous antibiotics started at 11.15 am with 100 ml of Meronem, which was followed by 100 ml of Zofran to protect my stomach from all the antibiotics I was taking. This was followed with 300 ml of Zetalid and 250 ml of Voncon, which finished at 1.30 pm.

I was able to rest in the afternoon before heading to the doctor for a 7 pm prostate PiezoWave.

At 7.30 pm I was back on the intravenous drip with the same cocktail as earlier in the day to fight the bacterial infection in my prostate. After three-and-a-half hours the intravenous session was over.

I had completed my seventh prostate injection and seventh intravenous antibiotics week.

## WEEK 24: Further prostate massages and agreeing final treatment plan.

### Monday 13 March

I didn't feel tired this Monday like I normally did after a prostate injection week. I took this as a good sign.

At 1 pm, I visited the doctor for my usual prostate massage, penis erection PiezoWave and prostate PiezoWave. I discussed my remaining treatment plan with the doctor, who was suggesting I have a three-week break from intravenous antibiotics. The go-forward plan was likely to be two prostate massages, two prostate PiezoWaves and one penis erection PiezoWave per day for the next three weeks. This would be followed up with an injection in four weeks' time.

It was nice to rest and relax in the afternoon before my second batch of treatment for the day at 9.30 pm. This was a prostate massage and prostate PiezoWave. The doctor and I also discussed the planned treatment plan over the next few weeks in more detail.

## Tuesday 14 March

I was at the doctor's clinic at 12.30 pm for my first appointment of the day.

While waiting for my appointment I talked to fellow patients Christos and Victor. (You can read their stories at the back of the book.) Again, it was shocking to hear how the symptoms of Chronic Prostatitis were also terrible for these poor sufferers.

The range of symptoms of Chronic Prostatitis I kept hearing about was becoming larger and larger.

At 1.30 pm I entered the doctor's treatment room for a prostate massage, penis erection PiezoWave and prostate PiezoWave.

I explained to the doctor how I was getting a different burning sensation in the tip of my penis and was needing to urinate very frequently this morning. The doctor said it was most likely the residue antibiotics from the injection last week leaving my prostatic ducts. I certainly hoped the staphylococcus aureus bacteria wasn't forming another army.

In the evening before my appointment, I had some great banter with fellow patients Nikos and Victor. Some weeks ago, I had nicknamed the doctor's surgery 'The Pleasure Palace'. Another patient, Panegotis, also cleverly named the clinic 'The Pressure Palace'.

Victor also came up with a very funny motto for the clinic: 'no pleasure without pressure'.

Jokes aside, the camaraderie and humour shared between patients, as well as the sharing of our personal stories, was a great help and motivation in getting through the program.

At 9.30 pm I did a prostate massage with heavy pressure from the doctor to break down any hard prostate tissue.

I almost regretted sharing the Spandau Ballet *I Don't Need This Pressure On* and Queen's *Under Pressure* with my friends as a pre-treatment joke.

After my prostate massage I also did a more relaxed prostate PiezoWave before heading to my accommodation to rest.

## Wednesday 15 March

I had a later 1.30 pm appointment today. The doctor started by pressing my prostate very vigorously and hard. It was one of the strongest prostate massages I had experienced so far. It was obvious the doctor was doing everything he could to dislodge any remaining bacterial colonies and sclerotic tissue in my prostate.

I then did an erection penis PiezoWave and prostate PiezoWave. I left the doctor's clinic feeling more tired than when I walked in, but I was now confident all the treatment was taking me in the right direction to getting my life back.

After an afternoon rest, I was back at the doctor's clinic – aka 'The Pleasure Palace' – at 8 pm for another prostate massage. The doctor was pressing hard again on my prostate and said he was resolving the final details. I also did a prostate PiezoWave which was a bit more relaxing.

## Thursday 16 March

My appointment was earlier today due to the doctor having prostate injection surgery on three patients mid-afternoon.

At 11 am I completed a very strong prostate massage followed by a penis erection PiezoWave and prostate PiezoWave. After my treatment I caught up with fellow patient Christos. It was really interesting to hear how Christos also tried to exercise through the symptoms of Chronic Prostatitis just like myself.

In the afternoon I had a nice rest before my evening appointment.

While waiting for my evening appointment I was feeling some burning in the tip of my penis. I really hoped it wasn't because I mistakenly ate some high-carbohydrate quinoa salad for breakfast. The doctor advised me it was most likely the residue antibiotic waste products that were still leaving my prostate glandular ducts.

This was one of the reasons he was currently pressing so hard on my prostate during this week's massages. The doctor was trying to flush out these waste products from my prostate. When they did exit my body, they caused some mild burning.

Following completion of my firm prostate massage and a more relaxing prostate PiezoWave, I was free to go to my room and rest.

## Friday 17 March

Before my doctor's appointment today I had to go to The Central Clinic of Athens to settle my €1050 outstanding invoice from my last intravenous week. Throughout the intravenous week you are charged a daily bed rate as well as for the cost of the antibiotic medications and treatment you consume.

It was then the short walk to the doctor's clinic for a 2 pm appointment. I did a prostate massage, penis erection PiezoWave and prostate PiezoWave. On the penis PiezoWave the doctor seemed to be pushing my erections even harder. The doctor said my erections were now in a very healthy and strong situation.

After an afternoon rest, I did another prostate massage and prostate PiezoWave in the evening.

## Saturday 18 March

I had not planned to go away this weekend due to the colder weather so the doctor arranged a full day of treatment for me.

At 11.30 am I had a very firm prostate massage. The doctor mentioned that I now did not sweat any more, even during very strong prostate massages. To him this was a very good sign and showed I had a healthy prostate with less stress on my neural system during the massage. The doctor explained when there is pain due to massaging the inflamed prostate, the pain causes the body to create adrenalin output and subsequent sweating.

The penis erection PiezoWave that followed was again extremely strong. It felt like the doctor was again testing my erection capacity to the maximum with the erection pumping device he placed on my penis. The prostate massage that followed was painless and more relaxed.

At 8.30 pm I finished off my week's treatment with another prostate massage and a prostate PiezoWave.

## WEEK 25: Prostate massages and prostate PiezoWaves to fix the final details.

### Monday 20 March

I started the week with a strong prostate massage at 1 pm. This was followed up with a piezo shockwave treatment on my erect penis and a PiezoWave up through my anal area towards my prostate. The doctor's focus was to smooth out any sclerotic tissue on my prostate where bacteria may be hiding.

I then had an afternoon rest before my evening appointment. At 8.30 pm I did another strong prostate massage and a more relaxed prostate PiezoWave.

## Tuesday 21 March

The doctor was very busy today, so I went into my appointment at 2 pm. The doctor and I talked again about how commitment is so important while doing the program. We discussed one patient who instead of coming for treatment every day would come every seven to ten days.

> The bottom line is if you do not fully believe in this program or cannot commit to it, you will stand no chance of eliminating the disease.

I had my prostate massage, penis erection PiezoWave and prostate PiezoWave.

I felt a little more tired than usual when I left the doctor's clinic, but overall, I felt in pretty good condition now.

In the evening before my appointment, I met a patient who had been fully treated by the program. He had become totally microbe free and had zero to one level leukocytes, which are the required level showing no bacteria is present.

This patient however became reinfected by a different microbe, most likely through having unprotected sex with his partner again. To me this demonstrated how important it was to keep up sexual protection and discipline after the program.

At 9 pm I did a prostate massage and prostate PiezoWave. My prostate was feeling strong and soft now.

## Wednesday 22 March

My first appointment today was at 4 pm due to a very busy doctor's clinic. I completed the usual prostate massage, penis erection PiezoWave and prostate PiezoWave treatment.

The doctor and I discussed the plans for my eighth prostate injection next week. We also discussed how important the antibiotic prostate injections are as a faster track to curing Chronic Prostatitis.

At 9 pm I did another prostate massage. It was a very challenging one as the doctor twirled and pressed his finger on the base of my urethra. The doctor said he could now access this area better as it was not now protected by fibrotic or sclerotic tissue. He said the tissue near my urethra was now more elastic, which meant he could access it and pressure it more easily.

It was as if he was discharging the very last infection from me when he pressed this area and I started to sweat during the massage for the first time in months. This particular prostate massage really sapped my energy and was tough to get through.

I followed this up with a prostate PiezoWave before some rest.

## Thursday 23 March

My regular treatment was at 2 pm today, consisting of the usual prostate massage to break down any final spots of sclerotic tissue or inflammation. I then had a penis erection PiezoWave to send shockwaves through my erect penis to promote better blood flow and rejuvenation.

My final morning treatment was prostate PiezoWave shockwaves triggered up through my anus towards my prostate to make all my prostate tissue as elastic and healthy as possible. The doctor said he was fixing the minor details now and wanted no areas where the bacteria could hide out.

I was now starting to look forward to at least a week off the treatment in a few weeks. I was reaching a critical juncture in the program where the next prostate scan and sperm test results would be crucially important.

I was really hoping to wrap everything up soon and be completely cured.

At 9 pm I did a prostate massage and prostate PiezoWave.

### Friday 24 March

I did a 1 pm prostate massage, penis erection PiezoWave and prostate PiezoWave. I still seemed to be getting some mild burning at the very tip of my penis I was not entirely happy about. I was not sure if it was the morning coffee I was drinking or some microbes still hanging around.

> Because I had been suffering symptoms so long it was becoming a struggle to know what was a normal bodily function down below and what was not.

The doctor said I should monitor this closely over the next few days.

In the evening I did a prostate massage and prostate PiezoWave, still with the nagging feeling I had some mild burning at the end of my penis.

## WEEK 26: Intraprostatic injection eight.

### Monday 27 March

I noticed when I awoke that the head of my penis was red with a type of fungal infection. I was not sure whether it was because of all the antibiotics I was taking or not. I mentioned this to the doctor at my 12.30 pm appointment and he suggested I apply Travogen cream twice a day.

I had my first prostate massage following a two-day break as well as a penis erection PiezoWave and prostate PiezoWave. The doctor then advised me my prostate injection would take place this coming Friday rather than the usual Thursday surgery. This was due to availability of some key staff in The Central Clinic of Athens operating theatre.

In the afternoon I checked out some new accommodation to move to as the hotel I was in was nearly doubling its prices due to the first tourists of the season starting to arrive.

At 9.30 pm I had a prostate massage and prostate PiezoWave treatment before heading back to get some good rest before my intravenous antibiotics started again.

## Tuesday 28 March

I started my intravenous antibiotics from 10.30 am. My cocktail to fight the remaining bacteria this time was:

### Morning

- Voncon 250 ml
- Meronem 100 ml
- Zyvoxid 300 ml
- Losec
- Zofran 4 ml

### Evening

- Voncon 250 ml
- Meronem 100 ml
- Zyvoxid 300 ml
- Zofran 4 ml mixed with saline

It took about two-and-a-half hours for the antibiotics to drip into my arm. Following this I did the short walk up to the doctor's clinic for my usual treatment of a prostate massage, penis erection PiezoWave and prostate PiezoWave.

After a nice afternoon's rest, I was back on the intravenous antibiotics at 8.30 pm. I finished the first two bottles in an hour before the doctor called me to go to his clinic. He wanted to do another transrectal scan on my prostate to get an accurate read of any inflammation before the intravenous antibiotics fully kicked in.

*My tenth transrectal prostate scan showed just one small dot of inflammation was remaining. It was located just under my urethra where it entered the prostate.*

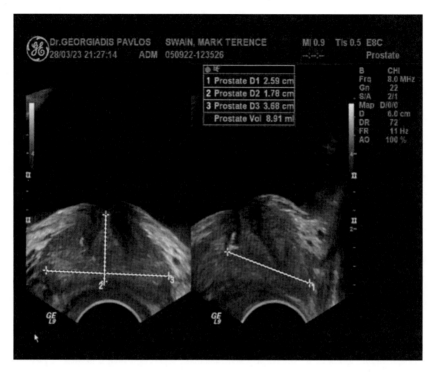

It was this small remaining area of bacteria and inflammation that was still causing me some extremely mild penile burning. The doctor seemed quite frustrated viewing this small red dot on my prostate that was left. I could see in his eyes he was now on a mission to terminate it.

After my transrectal scan I did a prostate massage where the focus was on this small red dot – the inflamed lower urethra area. I also did a prostate PiezoWave to trigger shockwaves into this small remaining area of inflammation.

With my probiotic tablets running low I stocked up on a new bottle from the doctor before heading back to The Central Clinic of Athens to finish my remaining two bottles of antibiotics between 10.30 pm and midnight.

## Wednesday 29 March

I started my intravenous antibiotics at 10 am. First I received a bottle of 4 ml of Zofran plus saline, followed by 100 ml of Meronem, 250 ml of Voncon and 300 ml of Zetalid.

These antibiotics finished at 1.15 pm and I was free to go to the doctor to do my twentieth uroflow test.

*My twentieth uroflow test showed my highest average flow rate to date at 20.1 ml per second and a high maximum flow rate of 30.1 ml per second.*

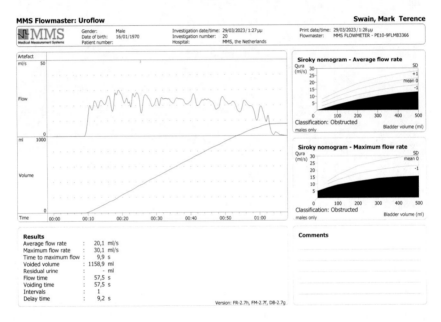

After the uroflow test I did a prostate massage, penis erection PiezoWave and prostate PiezoWave.

In the evening I started my antibiotics at 9 pm. Over one hour, the first two bottles slowly dripped into me. I then went to the doctor's clinic for a prostate massage, again focused heavily on my urethra, and a prostate PiezoWave.

I then went back to The Central Clinic of Athens intravenous therapy ward to continue my intravenous antibiotics between

10.30 pm and 1 am, finishing the remaining bottles of Voncon and Zetalid.

One interesting learning while taking the antibiotics today was when I spread my hand and fingers out widely, the antibiotics dripped into me faster and more efficiently. I was definitely going to use this technique moving forward.

## Thursday 30 March

I was at The Central Clinic of Athens at 11 am ready to have a new intravenous cannula inserted in a vein in my right arm. I had asked for the cannula in my left arm to be taken out last night so I could sleep better and wake more refreshed for an important work call.

After the antibiotics I went to the doctor's clinic for a prostate massage, penis erection PiezoWave and stronger and wider ranging prostate PiezoWave.

The doctor explained to me that from tomorrow he was going to change my intravenous medication and substitute the Zyvoxid/ Zetalid with Tycagil. I was not very pleased with this as I'd avoided Tycagil throughout my entire treatment program so far (Tycagil is one of the world's strongest antibiotics). Tycagil looks like dark yellow urine, and I'd seen it previously cause stomach cramps, nausea and rashes on the face.

The doctor however was insistent: now was the time to introduce Tycagil on the staphylococcus aureus remaining bacteria still present in and around where my lower urethra entered my prostate.

The goal was to go atomic and totally obliterate the remaining staphylococcus aureus bacteria.

The doctor explained he had seen very positive results deploying Tycagil on other patients at the end of their treatment.

After a solid lunch at Nikitas restaurant, I rested in the afternoon before my next intravenous session at The Central Clinic of Athens.

At 7.30 pm I started my evening bottles of intravenous antibiotics which flowed very quickly into a new vein in my left arm about 7 cm down from the elbow. At 9.30 pm I was finished on the night's antibiotics and free to go to the doctor for a prostate massage and prostate PiezoWave to round out the day.

> Tomorrow would be my first encounter with the dreaded Tycagil antibiotics and my eighth prostate injection. I rested early to get ready for the big day ahead.

## Friday 31 March

I visited the doctor at 10 am for my normal prostate massage, penis erection PiezoWave and prostate PiezoWave. It was then down to The Central Clinic of Athens to start my intravenous antibiotic cocktail. I started at 11 am and finished at 2.30 pm, shortly before the surgery was planned. The Tycagil quickly gave me a bit of a headache and red, dry-skinned cheeks on my face.

As soon as I had pretty much finished the antibiotics a senior nurse from the operating theatre called me and two fellow patients, George and Doru, down to the operating theatre. I was glad I had quickly slipped into my hospital-style operating gown as soon as the antibiotics stopped.

The three of us walked with the senior nurse in our blue gowns down to the operating theatre level. I was very quickly put on a hospital bed trolley and covered in a blanket; it was time for business again.

*All ready for my eighth prostate injection. I was hoping and praying this would be my last one.*

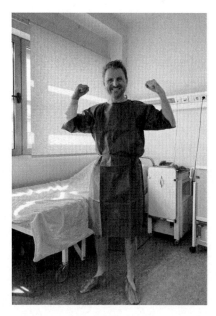

I had blood taken out of my left arm that would be used in my penis PRP rejuvenation injection. The full procedure ahead of me was:

- Urethra dilation (to widen my urethra and increase urine flow).

- Fibrinolytic agent injection (to stimulate tissue repair in the penis).

- Intraprostatic injection (to target the remaining bacteria and inflammation in my lower prostate near the connection with my urethra). The complete mixture of antibiotics to be injected in my prostate included Tycagil, Meronem, Mefoxil, Voncon, Zithromax, Ciproxin and Zyvoxid.

- PRP penis injection (to stimulate blood flow and vessels in the penile shaft).

- PRP prostate injection (to help with increased prostate healing).

Once again, I was wheeled into the operating room where anaesthetic was slowly applied so surgery could start.

Once I came around from the surgery, I stayed in the recovery room next to the operating theatre for twenty minutes. I was then wheeled on a hospital trolley bed back to the intravenous therapy ward where my fellow patients also shortly followed me like zombies. We were all a bit dazed and tired. Injection eight for me however was complete.

I waited over an hour before I took the gauze bandage out of my backside. My urination due to the penis dilatation was very painful, and generally I felt a bit exhausted.

In the evening I did just a prostate PiezoWave at 8.30 pm, before more intravenous antibiotics between 9 and 11.30 pm.

## Saturday 1 April

I started my antibiotics between 10.30 and 11.00 am before the doctor called me to go to his clinic. I quickly asked a nurse to disconnect my cannula and I walked up to the doctor's clinic for a penis erection PiezoWave and strong prostate PiezoWave. A prostate massage was not on the menu today following yesterday's prostate injection.

The doctor said he had injected my prostate very well yesterday and he expected no microbes to be left. From 12.30 to 3.30 pm I went back on the antibiotics, finishing my 250 ml of Voncon, 100 ml of Meronem and 100 ml of Tycagil.

With a bit of dizziness and stomach gurgling due to the Tycagil, I went for lunch at my go-to restaurant Nikitas. Given my antibiotics were running late today I didn't even go to my room to rest; I went straight back to the hospital to lay on my bed to relax for two hours before my next appointment with the doctor.

At 6.50 pm I did a quick prostate PiezoWave.

I was feeling really tired by now from all the antibiotics. I nearly fell asleep on the doctor's treatment table.

At 7.15 pm I started my intravenous antibiotics with 100 ml of Meronem, 250 ml of Voncon, 100 ml of Tycagil and 4 ml of diluted Zofran.

My antibiotics finished at 9.45 pm and I was free. I was however noticing a specific pain in my left flank. It was in an area which was one of my original symptom problem areas. I definitely wanted to find out what this was when I spoke with the doctor in the morning.

### Sunday 2 April

I visited the doctor at 11 am to do a quick prostate PiezoWave. I mentioned to him about the specific very focused pain in my left flank. The doctor explained to me it was because Thursday's injection in my prostate had helped release the nerve to my iliopsoas muscle.

I found this amazing as this was always one of the main sources of my pain before the program even started. The fact that an injection in my prostate could release the long-standing pressure pain point in my left flank amazed me.

From 11.30 am till 2.30 pm I finished my four bottles of antibiotics and went to lunch with fellow patients Doru and George. We were all very relieved to disconnect our cannulas and to have gotten through a big, demanding prostate injection week.

## WEEK 27: Post-injection prostate massaging and monitoring. Resumption of oral antibiotics.

### Monday 3 April

The doctor's prostate massage on me at 1 pm had a strong focus on my urethra to spread last week's injected antibiotics around my prostate as much as possible. The doctor was doing everything he could to ensure 100% of bacterial microbes were killed.

After the prostate massage I did a penis erection PiezoWave and prostate PiezoWave.

I told the doctor I was still feeling very tired from last week's antibiotics, particularly the Tycagil, but otherwise I felt fine. I went home after the treatment to cook a huge steak and vegetable stir-fry with olive oil to help me recharge.

Before my 9 pm appointment I obtained a list of antibiotics that went into my prostate last week. There was Tycagil, Meronem, Mefoxil, Voncon, Zithromax, Ciproxin and Zyvoxid.

I then had a prostate massage where the doctor focused heavily on the centre of my prostate and urethra area to again fully disperse any residue antibiotics to every corner in my prostate.

I then did a prostate PiezoWave to round out the day.

## Tuesday 4 April

I visited the doctor at 1 pm for a prostate massage, again with the focus on the centre of my prostate and the area where the urethra meets the prostate. The massage and finger movement on my prostate was quite difficult to take after last week's injection. I also had a penis erection PiezoWave and prostate PiezoWave.

At 9.30 pm I had another prostate massage focused on the urethra area and a more powerful prostate PiezoWave. The machine's waves now had a higher piezo strength that could transfer electromagnetic signals up to 3 cm into my prostate.

I came home in a taxi with fellow patient and taxi driver Giovanni.

## Wednesday 5 April

I visited the doctor at 1 pm for another swirling, strong prostate and urethra massage. This was followed by my usual PiezoWave treatments.

The PiezoWave used this morning was a different version again that projected waves up to 2 cm into my prostate. The doctor was still trying to break down any lurking hard tissue in my prostate.

I had my next appointment at 9 pm. I met many of the regular patients at the doctor's clinic including George, Thomas, Panegotis, Alexander and John.

It was time for another twirling prostate massage focused on my urethra at 9.15 pm, which was quite painful and made me sweat. This was followed up with a prostate PiezoWave.

## Thursday 6 April

I had an earlier appointment with the doctor at 11 am today as he had surgery at 2 pm. I had another prostate massage with a heavy focus again on where my urethra met my prostate.

This was followed up with a penis erection PiezoWave where my penis literally stood up like a tent pole. The doctor seemed very pleased with this.

I then had a more relaxing prostate PiezoWave.

On the way back to my hotel, I picked up some Sporanox tablets for my intermittent penis fungal infection and also weighed myself.

*I was now weighing in at 68 kg with clothes on, some 10.5 kg less than when I started the program.*

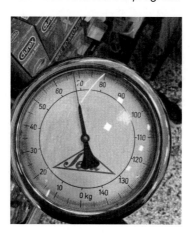

After an afternoon of rest, I was back at the doctor's surgery for my 9 pm appointment. The doctor explained to me how some patients also have bacteria that enters and lives in their sinuses. Often the male has gone 'down under' to pleasure the female and picked up some unwanted bugs that make a home in the cosy cave of the sinuses.

Luckily for me my sinuses were fine, so I proceeded to have my regular strong prostate massage, which although very strong, was easy to take because it wasn't so focused on my urethra. I also had a ten-minute prostate PiezoWave.

## Friday 7 April

I had my first appointment at 1 pm. The doctor advised me that after today he was taking me off the tablet antibiotics Norocin and Augmentin. He wanted me to have a twenty-day or so break from the antibiotics before performing my next sperm culture test to check bacterial status in my prostate.

I had a prostate massage, which even under very strong pressure was easy. This was followed by a penis erection PiezoWave and prostate PiezoWave.

In the evening I had a prostate massage at 9.30 pm. I asked the doctor what he was focusing on during the massage and he said it was to push any remaining microbes out of my prostate.

I was a bit surprised by this as I thought last week's injection would have killed them all. The doctor said if there were any remaining microbes left amongst the residue antibiotic fluids he had injected, he wanted to flush them all out.

The doctor explained I would come off the antibiotics tonight and I should carefully monitor any symptoms over the coming days.

I then did a prostate PiezoWave before I was free.

## Saturday 8 April

From today I stopped taking my regular antibiotics. It felt a bit weird as I was so used to the routine of taking them that I reached for my medicine bag and nearly took them out of habit.

I would have sixteen days antibiotic free before my next sperm sample was analysed for harmful bacteria.

I did a 10.30 am appointment with the doctor who completed a very hard prostate massage which was no problem for me. I did a penis erection PiezoWave, which I explained to the doctor was like drinking a daily cappuccino for me now.

> I now had no thoughts of women or sex or any penis pain when this penis erectile treatment was done.

I also did a relaxing prostate PiezoWave while lying on my side on the doctor's leather treatment table.

I was free to rest in the afternoon before my final appointment of the week. At 7 pm I did a prostate massage and prostate PiezoWave.

Fellow patient Doru explained to me that the doctor was visited two days ago by a former patient, Omar, who was fully cured some four years ago. This was reassuring to hear as I was starting to have some doubts about whether a complete and full cure of Chronic Prostatitis was possible.

## WEEK 28: Antibiotic-free treatment week before Easter break.

### Monday 10 April

My first meeting of the new week was at 1 pm in the doctor's Central Athens clinic. I had my usual prostate massage, penis erection PiezoWave and prostate PiezoWave treatments.

I explained to the doctor my energy levels felt much better now I was off the antibiotic tablets. He was not surprised by this and said my body was in a much stronger position to bounce back now.

After an afternoon rest and healthy meal, I was back in the doctor's clinic for my evening appointment. I explained to the doctor again just before my 8.30 pm prostate massage how my energy levels were feeling so much better since I came off the antibiotics. The doctor mentioned this is expected and with my healthier prostate I would now recover much more quickly and get a big boost in energy levels.

## The prostate is the main energy source for men and a healthy prostate generally means good energy levels.

After my evening prostate massage, I did a prostate PiezoWave to round out the day.

### Tuesday 11 April

During my 1 pm appointment I had a prostate massage, penis erection PiezoWave and prostate PiezoWave as usual. I mentioned to the doctor I was getting some burning and a weird sensation on my penis head and urethra. The doctor recommended I go back on the Sporanox tablets for a few days and closely monitor the situation. I was hoping and praying the microbes were not rearming with me now off the antibiotic tablets.

In the evening I returned to the doctor for another appointment where I had a prostate massage and prostate PiezoWave. I was now really starting to look forward to my ten-day break from treatment over the Easter holidays in Greece.

## Wednesday 12 April

At 2 pm I had a prostate massage, which despite being very heavy pressure and strong movement on my urethra by the doctor was relatively easy to manage. I then had a penis erection PiezoWave and prostate PiezoWave. The afternoon was free for me to rest before my evening appointment.

At 9 pm I had a prostate massage with a focused twirling on my urethra. The doctor said my prostate was soft, spongy and healthy. It was a stark contrast to the calcified hard prostate feeling when I arrived in Athens.

The prostate PiezoWave was no problem, and caused a slight sensation at the end of my penis, likely from the release of more small, blocked nerves, which was a good thing.

I now had just one more day of treatment before my break.

## Thursday 13 April

During my appointment today at 12.30 pm I explained to the doctor how Chronic Prostatitis used to cause me so much tiredness and lethargy.

Even simple tasks like shopping and trying on clothes were exhausting and a real struggle.

I recalled one time after shopping for around two hours how I returned home absolutely exhausted and unable to do anything for the rest of the day. For me this was debilitating as I had always been very fit and able to do short triathlons and play tennis for three or four hours without issues.

The doctor performed a prostate massage, penis erection, PiezoWave and prostate PiezoWave on me before I went back to my apartment to relax.

In the early evening at 6.30 pm, I had a firm prostate massage and final prostate PiezoWave before I was free to go on vacation.

## Friday 14 April

It was great to head off to Turkey for my nine-night holiday. One thing I noticed now while travelling was the increased energy I had. I also found that my ears were easier to clear when I landed from a flight compared to before. For some reason Chronic Prostatitis previously caused my ears, particularly my right ear, to block, even when I wasn't flying.

> I was feeling by now a more confident, fitter and stronger person.

I was determined to really relax and recharge my batteries on this holiday, particularly following the constant daily treatment and antibiotics I had been undergoing.

## Ten-day Easter break from the program and off all antibiotics

It was so good to have a break from the program. I had arranged to go to Turkey, as my Greek Visa was expiring and I wanted to go to a destination that was close by, where the weather was nice and I could relax.

My plan was to have ten days resting, relaxing, eating good food, building up some gentle gym exercise and playing some golf.

> One immediate thing I noticed on the holiday was I was waking up early and felt invigorated to do things.

I would wake up naturally between 6 and 7 am each day and head straight to the hotel swimming pool. As the first swimmer of the day, I generally had the pool to myself and would do twenty lengths.

It was nice not having to think about when I would take my antibiotic tablets or what time I should leave each day to visit the doctor's clinic. I really felt like my old self again, and had high energy back out on the golf course. Before my treatment started, eighteen holes of golf exhausted me and during one period my back was in so much pain, I could not even pick the ball up out of the hole.

> The sun, great diet, gentle stretching in the gym, light weights, swimming and golf really did me a power of good. The ten-day break was what my body and mind had been craving.

## WEEK 29: Fourth sperm test and recommencement of daily prostate treatment.

### Monday 24 April

It was a real shock to the system flying back to Athens and getting ready for my first appointment back. At 11.30 am I did a penis erection PiezoWave followed by a normal prostate PiezoWave. The doctor then gloved up to give me a prostate massage. Surprisingly, the prostate massage was very easy to take after my ten-day break and my prostate felt very soft and spongy.

This would be the prostate pressure massage before my fourth sperm test.

Following my massage, I headed off with fellow patient Christos to the Mycolab clinic where we would both need to deposit our sperm sample. It was nice of Christos to offer me a lift and we had some good mutual patient banter on the way there.

*The setting for my fourth sperm test was the same.*

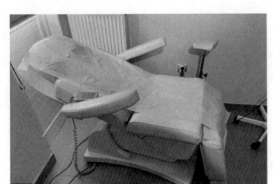

I found it a juggling act trying to manoeuvre myself to the point of ejaculation without dropping either my sperm bottle or mobile tuned into the erotic website of my choice.

Many aspects of my sperm were going to be analysed in this €320 test, including a complete sperm diagram, bacteria and white blood cell count.

In the late afternoon I started back on the Augmentin and Norocin antibiotics as per the doctor's request. Unfortunately, or fortunately, the doctor came down with a cold this afternoon so my evening appointment was cancelled. I was quite relieved as I was still a bit tired from yesterday's travel and felt like I was shaking off some kind of cold bug myself.

Instead of visiting the doctor I chilled out and went to bed early.

## Tuesday 25 April

I had an 11 am appointment with the doctor today to do a prostate massage, penis PiezoWave and prostate PiezoWave. The prostate massage was very easy to take, and when the doctor asked me if I still had any sensitive areas I mentioned there was possibly some sensitivity still near my urethra. I did mention that I also had some slight pain in my penis from a cut on my foreskin that came out during or just after yesterday's strong penis erection PiezoWave treatment. A slight cut had appeared on my penis shaft where the foreskin meets the penis head and it was annoyingly painful.

The doctor did another very small injection in the base of my penis to send the blood flow there and proceeded to carry out today's erection suction machine treatment followed by a penis PiezoWave. My holiday was really starting to feel like a distant memory!

This was followed by a prostate PiezoWave with his new prostate PiezoWave machine, which could send signals 6 cm up towards my prostate. I was free to rest and relax in the afternoon in my new AirBnb apartment, which was a very convenient ten-minute walk from the doctor's clinic.

In the evening I did a prostate massage and prostate PiezoWave at 7 pm to round out my treatment for the day.

## Wednesday 26 April

During my doctor's appointment at 11 am the sperm result relating to my white blood cell count came back from the microbiological laboratory Mycolab.

The leukocyte figure, if above one, shows your body is still fighting an infection. In other words, no microbes may be found on a sperm microbiological analysis, but if leukocytes are high this indicates bacteria are still likely present with the body's white blood cells fighting against it.

The doctor asked me when I last ejaculated and I said I hadn't for several weeks. This made the doctor feel the reading still had residue leukocytes from prior sperm build up and he suggested I may be best to do a fresh sperm test in two days. He said that given my lack of symptoms, my leukocyte reading was not expected to be above four.

After discussing the leukocyte reading with me, the doctor did a prostate massage on me and asked if it caused any burning or irritation. I replied I didn't think so.

*My sperm test two days ago showed that my white blood cell count*
*(leukocytes) was still showing 12 to 15 per field. This was much*
*higher than the 2 to 3 per field the doctor was expecting.*

Ιδιωτικό Διαγνωστικό Εργαστήριο Ειδικών Λοιμώξεων - Μυκητιάσεων & Μικροβιολογικών Εξετάσεων
• Τμήμα Βιοπαθολογίας (Ορμονολογικό-Βιοχημικό-Αιματολογικό-Ανοσολογικό) - Μοριακής Βιολογίας - Προγεννητικού Ελέγχου
• Τμήμα Κυτταρολογίας - Εργαστήριο Ψηφιακής Ανάλυσης Εικόνας
(Digital Image Analysis Lab)

Λεωφ. Κηφισίας 354 Χαλάνδρι Τ.Κ. 15233
ΑΦΜ:998012799 - ΔΟΥ: ΧΑΛΑΝΔΡΙΟΥ
Τηλ. 210-8028817, 210-6890505 Φαξ; 210-6890506
www.mycolab.gr - info@mycolab.gr

| | | |
|---|---|---|
| Patient name: | MARK SWAIN | DATE: 24/04/2023 |

### CULTURE OF SPERM

Leukocytes (White Blood Cells):    Few (12-15) per field
Stem Fungus:
Neisser:
Gramm stain:

**Cultivation (aerobic)**

**Cultivation (anaerobic)**

**Chamydiaceae:**

**Mycoplasma Fermentans**

**Mycoplasma Hominis:**

**Ureaplasma Urealyticum:**

**COMMENTS**
pH 8.0 - Hb (+) Erythrocytes Few ( 8-10) per field

I then had a penis erection PiezoWave and prostate PiezoWave treatment. In a way I was happy to be doing a fresh sperm test in two days to get a second reading.

In the evening I had a prostate massage and prostate PiezoWave. The doctor and I discussed my sperm result again with the higher than expected leukocyte reading. We discussed whether the fact I had a cold may be affecting the result. The doctor explained there was a possibility a virus infection from a cold may have some effect on the reading, but the doctor was leaning towards some left over residue from a few weeks ago containing previous leukocytes still being in my sperm.

We agreed to proceed with a retest and to check the data that would come back.

## Thursday 27 April

My first task of the morning was to undertake a uroflow test. Despite drinking many glasses of water this morning, a coffee and a tea, I did not have a full bladder. I'd made the mistake of urinating when I got up.

My uroflow test showed a low volume of only around 250 ml. This was less than a quarter of what I normally gave as a sample and was not enough to determine how efficient my urinary flow currently was.

The doctor said I should come back in the evening and do a new urine sample with a larger volume. Next up, I did a transrectal ultrasound on my prostate. I was literally praying for a clean result with no inflammation after all I'd been through.

I was gutted. My urethra still showed a very minor red spot of inflammation, which indicated microbes were still present.

I explained to the doctor that my urine flow had not been overly strong during my recent ten-day break. The doctor mentioned that even a small oedema on the urethra can cause restriction to the urinary flow.

*My eleventh transrectal scan still showed a very small
red dot at the lower centre of my urethra.*

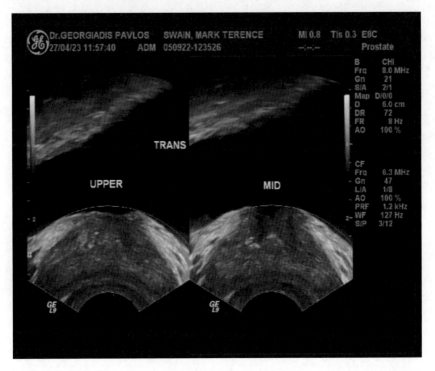

All this new information put me in a dilemma about what to
do next. I had to be in Singapore the week after next on 9 May to
deliver an important sales training course.

I had a prostate massage, penis PiezoWave and prostate PiezoWave
before walking out of the doctor's clinic somewhat dazed. To say
I was disappointed with still seeing inflammation on the transrectal
prostate scan would be an understatement.

It was starting to look like I would need to fly
back to Athens for more treatment after my trip to
Singapore, given the staphylococcus aureus still
seemed to be hanging around.

The doctor and I agreed to think about the future treatment options and discuss later in the day.

After a rest to shake off my worsening cold, I started drinking copious amounts of water before my evening appointment. At 8 pm I was ready, in fact desperate, to do my uroflow test and was almost struggling to walk due to the fullness of my bladder.

*My twenty-second uroflow test delivered my highest maximum flow rate to date of 32.6 ml per second. This was achieved from a relatively large quantity of 1.34 litres of bladder fluid.*

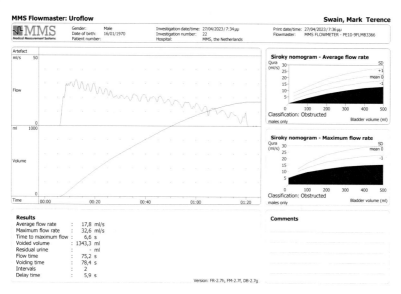

I then had a prostate massage and prostate PiezoWave. The doctor said he wanted to see my full microbiological sperm analysis results (not just the leukocytes) before deciding on his plan for tackling the stubborn remaining inflammation in my urethra.

## Friday 28 April

With my cold getting better I walked the short ten-minute stroll from my apartment in Neofytou Vamva street to the doctor's clinic. I was really tired kneeling down for my prostate massage but took it without much pain.

It felt like my prostate was starting to get tired and sensitive again due to the twice-daily pressure sessions. I had the penis erection piezo treatment with shock waves sent through it over about twenty minutes and finished with a prostate PiezoWave.

## By now I knew the doctor so well, I held the prostate PiezoWave machine against my anal area while he took an urgent phone call.

My entire morning treatment was done in about forty-five minutes and I was free to rest for the afternoon.

It was so much better being close to the doctor's clinic from a convenience point of view during treatment, compared to other places I had stayed at. This however was not always possible with Central Athens accommodation increasing in scarcity and price as we moved into the tourist season.

In the evening at 8.30 pm I had a prostate massage and prostate PiezoWave. I said to the doctor I was feeling a bit down due to my cold and yesterday's transrectal scan on my prostate that still showed urethra inflammation. The doctor explained I was so close to the end of the program and I should stay positive. He even said the microbes could be sending signals to my endocrine system making me feel negative and wanting to give up.

I walked out of the doctor's clinic with a renewed determination to see this project through and conquer the staphylococcus aureus microbes.

### Saturday 29 April

I visited the doctor at 10.15 am. I explained to him that I was focusing all my body's energy towards my urethra to kill the remaining microbes. The doctor said this was a very good idea as mindset is crucial to overcome the deceptive powers of the microbes. I was feeling more positive again and was determined to work with the doctor to fully complete this job.

I had a prostate massage, penis erection PiezoWave and prostate PiezoWave treatment between 10.15 and 11 am. I left the doctor with more of a spring in my step and a renewed determination to win my battle over Chronic Prostatitis. I had an evening prostate massage and prostate PiezoWave and was done for the week.

## WEEK 30: Daily prostate massages and prostate PiezoWaves while awaiting sperm analysis results. Targeting the final small red dot of prostate inflammation.

### Monday 1 May

The doctor very kindly came in to provide treatment to me today despite it being a public holiday. To me this demonstrated the fantastic commitment the doctor had to his patients' recovery.

At 10.30 am I had a prostate massage. I explained to the doctor that when he did the most aggressive massage and made side-to-side movements on the furthest point of my urethra, there was possibly still some burning or irritation.

I then had a penis erection PiezoWave followed by a prostate massage. I was then free to walk to my apartment on near-deserted streets to do some reading and work before my evening appointment.

At 7.30 pm I visited the doctor again for another hard and twirling urethra-focused finger prostate massage. I was feeling like the last of the microbes were steadily being pushed out of my urethra. The prostate massage was followed by a more relaxed prostate PiezoWave, before I was free to rest for the evening.

### Tuesday 2 May

I had my first prostate massage of the day at 1.30 pm. Again, the doctor twirled his right forefinger on my urethra to try to push out any last remaining microbes. I said to the doctor that I felt this strategy was working as I needed to urinate with some very slight burning sensation right after the massage.

I then had a penis erection PiezoWave treatment. It seemed that the doctor turned his pump erection machine up to its highest level possible. I jokingly said to him to be careful as he might break the machine and explode my precious manhood. I then took ten minutes of piezo shockwave on my erect penis to continue promoting healthy blood flow before a more relaxed prostate PiezoWave.

I had a later evening appointment at 9 pm, where again the prostate massage triggered a need to urinate and some mild burning sensation. I was unsure whether this was me psychologically wanting to rid myself of the last microbes or not. My day was rounded out with a prostate massage, which was no problem.

## Wednesday 3 May

I attended the doctor's clinic at 12.30 pm. Firstly I had a prostate massage done.

I was still awaiting the sperm analysis results from last week's test. The doctor therefore wanted to see if I had any symptoms associated with having microbes left while we awaited the official sperm results.

I said to the doctor that maybe there was a small sensitivity in the end of my urethra near the prostate, where the tissue did not feel so soft.

I then had a penis erection PiezoWave with the doctor's pump machine; again it was operating at a maximum level that was making me grit my teeth as I got harder and harder. Once I had reached a full erection the doctor did ten minutes of shockwave treatment on my penis. This was followed by a much more relaxing prostate PiezoWave.

In the evening at 8.30 I had another twirling prostate massage and a prostate PiezoWave.

## Thursday 4 May

This morning my long-awaited sperm results came through. It was not the reading I wanted; staphylococcus aureus bacteria were still present. This number was down from the original 80,000 cfu/ml number.

*My fourth sperm test showed 3,000 cfu/ml of staphylococcus aureus bacteria still present.*

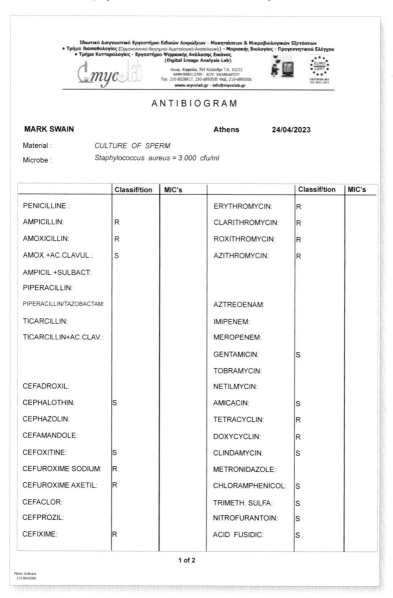

Ιδιωτικό Διαγνωστικό Εργαστήριο Ειδικών Λοιμώξεων - Μυκητιάσεων & Μικροβιολογικών Εξετάσεων
• Τμήμα Βιοπαθολογίας (Ορμονολογικό-Βιοχημικό-Αιματολογικό-Ανοσολογικό) - Μοριακής Βιολογίας - Προγεννητικού Ελέγχου
• Τμήμα Κυτταρολογίας - Εργαστήριο Ψηφιακής Ανάλυσης Εικόνας
(Digital Image Analysis Lab)

Λεωφ. Κηφισίας 354 Χαλάνδρι Τ.Κ. 15233
ΑΦΜ:998012799 - ΔΟΥ: ΧΑΛΑΝΔΡΙΟΥ
Τηλ. 210-8028817, 210-6890505 Φαξ: 210-6890506
www.mycolab.gr - info@mycolab.gr

Patient name:          MARK SWAIN                                      DATE:        24/04/2023

## CULTURE OF SPERM

Leukocytes (White Blood Cells):     Few (12-15) per field

Stem Fungus:

Neisser:

Gramm stain:

**Cultivation (aerobic)**

**Cultivation (anaerobic)**

**Chamydiaceae:**

**Mycoplasma Fermentans**

**Mycoplasma Hominis:**

**Ureaplasma Urealyticum:**

COMMENTS

pH  8.0 -  Hb (+) Erythrocytes Few ( 8-10) per field

The Doctor

The fact the staphylococcus aureus was still present in my prostate, despite my eight prostate injections and eight months on a very strict no-sugar and low-carbohydrate diet, was something I was starting to find surreal and terribly annoying.

I discussed these results with the doctor, who said ideally I needed to fly back from my work trip to Singapore next week to complete another prostate injection and finish the job.

I had a prostate massage, penis erection PiezoWave and prostate PiezoWave.

I was a bit down with my sperm result reading, but I really knew deep down with some of my lingering symptoms of mild burning and a sensitive urethra tissue that bacteria would still be present.

In the evening I had a prostate massage and prostate PiezoWave at 9 pm.

## Friday 5 May

At 11.30 am I visited the doctor to do a twirling prostate massage, penis erection PiezoWave and prostate PiezoWave.

I discussed my amazement with the doctor that microbial bacteria were still alive and present despite all I'd been through. The doctor said fighting the microbes was like fighting a smart alien army. He did however say once the bacteria count was below 10,000 cfu/ml he was confident he could eliminate them. I certainly hoped so.

In the evening at 9 pm I had another strong prostate massage and prostate PiezoWave.

### Saturday 6 May

At 9.30 am the doctor did an extremely strong prostate massage on me before my work trip to Singapore. He also did a penis erection PiezoWave which pushed my erection to the absolute maximum.

This was followed by a more sedate prostate PiezoWave.

I was now free to depart for five days before coming back next Friday to get prepared for intraprostatic injection nine the following week.

> I was hoping my next trip back to Greece would be my last, except for vacations.

## WEEK 31: Break from treatment for a business trip. Two days of prostate massages to get ready for another prostate injection.

During my five days off treatment for a business trip, I was feeling very strong and positive. I was simply amazed how well I could do my work and how creative my mind was.

Despite limited sleep in Singapore, I was able to deliver a very effective banking sales workshop and had energy to spare. Before my treatment, my work was badly affected to the point I did not have the energy to be creative or to deliver workshops without getting exhausted.

My trip away gave me a good taste of what life would be like when the Chronic Prostatitis treatment program was complete. But for now, I had to head back to Athens for one final push to fully eradicate the disease.

## Friday 12 May

On arrival back in Athens I went straight from the airport to a 12.30 pm meeting with the doctor, who by now I was calling 'Goldfinger'. I was soon undergoing a prostate massage again. I asked the doctor if my prostate felt the same as when I left Athens six days ago and he said yes.

He explained because my staphylococcus aureus microbial bacteria load was very low at 3,000 cfu/ml, there had been no deterioration of my prostate off the antibiotics and daily treatment during the last week.

I followed up the prostate massage with a penis erection PiezoWave and prostate PiezoWave.

I then stocked up on Norocin and Augmentin antibiotics so I could start immediately taking them again. The doctor wanted oral antibiotics to start complementing the daily prostate massages and PiezoWaves I would be having.

In the evening I had a prostate massage and prostate PiezoWave before retiring to try to get some sleep despite my jetlag.

## Saturday 13 May

After a great night's sleep recovering from my long trip back to Athens from Singapore, I was back at the doctor's at 11.30 am.

I had a prostate massage, penis erection PiezoWave and prostate PiezoWave over the next forty-five minutes.

### I explained to the doctor how alert and dynamic I was feeling doing day-to-day tasks.

I was thinking more clearly and positively in all my daily activities.

At 6 pm I had another prostate massage and prostate PiezoWave while still struggling with my jetlag. I joked with the doctor that

213

I may be the first ever patient to fall asleep during a prostate massage, but sadly that was not the case!

After my treatment I was free to rest for the remainder of the weekend. Next week would be intraprostatic injection week nine, so I needed to be rested and ready.

## WEEK 32: Week of intravenous antibiotics and intraprostatic prostate injection nine.

### Monday 15 May

My first task was to get a COVID-19 test done at The Central Clinic of Athens to confirm I was all clear to start my intravenous antibiotics there tomorrow.

At 1 pm I did a strong prostate massage, penis erection PiezoWave and prostate PiezoWave. The doctor's assistant gave me a list of the daily intravenous antibiotics I would be taking from tomorrow, which were:

### Morning

- 250 ml Voncon
- 100 ml Meronem
- 300 ml Zyvoxid
- 4 ml Zofran mixed with saline plus Losec

### Evening

- 250 ml Voncon
- 100 ml Meronem
- 300 ml Zyvoxid
- 4 ml Zofran mixed with saline

After my treatment this morning I rested in the afternoon before my 9.45 pm appointment with the doctor, where I had a prostate massage and prostate PiezoWave.

It was then time to get some sleep before the intravenous anti-biotics started tomorrow.

## Tuesday 16 May

I started my intravenous antibiotics at The Central Clinic of Athens at 9.45 am. The four bottles of fluid dripped into my arm very quickly over the next one-and-a-half hours.

Interestingly, after thirty minutes on the intravenous antibiotics I felt some nerve tingling in the end of my penis and in my prostate. I was convinced the antibiotics were hitting the final remaining inflammation and infection. After my first batch of antibiotics, I visited the doctor's clinic. There I completed another uroflow test.

*My twenty-third uroflow test showed a maximum urine flow of 30.8 ml per second. The doctor was content with this but not delighted. He said some form of urinary restriction was still present.*

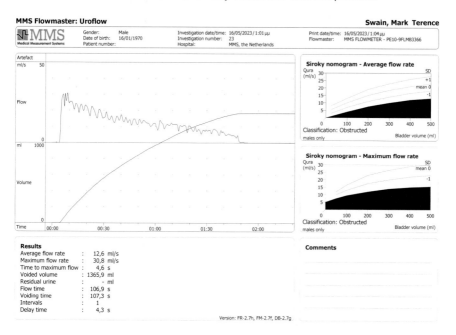

I then did my twelfth transrectal ultrasound scan.

*My twelfth transrectal scan still showed some very mild
inflammation at the tip of my urethra just before the end.*

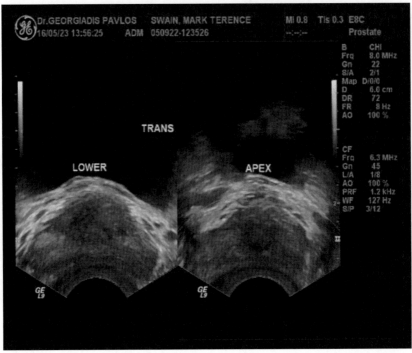

The doctor said this scan was better than the last one as the inflammation was only at the upper level. The doctor said he was confident he could shoot this point with his antibiotic injection cocktail this coming Thursday.

Following these tests I had a prostate massage, penis erection PiezoWave and prostate PiezoWave. I was already becoming tired from the intravenous antibiotics starting to take effect when I left the doctor's clinic at 2.30 pm.

At 6.30 pm I was back at The Central Clinic of Athens for two-and-a-half hours more of intravenous antibiotics. I then went to the doctor for a prostate massage and prostate PiezoWave at 10 pm. (If you have not worked it out yet, Dr Pavlos Georgiadis works incredibly hard. In fact, he is undoubtedly the hardest working person I have ever met.)

I said to the doctor during my prostate PiezoWave after the prostate massage that it felt as if the remaining slightly blocked area of my urethra was clearing. This was confirmed by my stronger urination when I left the treatment room. I was really starting to feel like I was on the home straight now, to finish this program and eliminate the Chronic Prostatitis disease.

## Wednesday 17 May

I was back on the intravenous antibiotics from 9.15 am until 11.45 am. This was followed by treatment from the doctor from 2 till 3 pm. I explained to the doctor before my prostate massage that it felt like something had really cleared in my urethra as I did not need to strain to force my initial urination like I usually did.

The prostate massage was followed up with a penis erection PiezoWave and prostate PiezoWave.

From 6.45 pm to 8.45 pm I completed my intravenous antibiotics. During my fourth bottle I noticed a sharp nerve pain in the end of my penis as if the medicine was really hitting the required spot on my lower urethra which controls these nerves.

It was then straight to the doctor, who did an evening prostate massage and prostate PiezoWave on me.

## Thursday 18 May

I had a very light breakfast of boiled eggs and avocado, given it was surgery day. Between 8.45 am and 10.15 am I took on board three bottles of intravenous antibiotics at the Central Clinic.

I then went to the doctor for a pre-surgery prostate massage, penis erection PiezoWave and prostate PiezoWave.

By noon I was back in The Central Clinic of Athens treatment room to finish my last morning bottle of antibiotics and get ready for my planned 2 pm surgery.

*My bed in The Central Clinic of Athens intravenous antibiotics therapy room.*

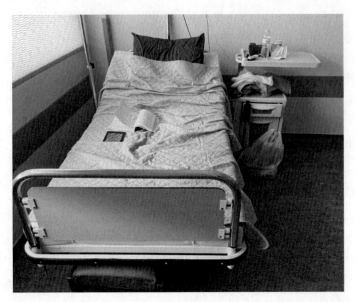

At 2.30 pm I was taken down to the operating theatre area for my intraprostatic injection.

My fellow patient George from Germany had his injection before me. At 3.30 pm I had blood taken out of my left arm for my PRP penis injection. I was then given anaesthetic in my right arm cannula to knock me out for the surgery. The summary of the surgery I would be undergoing was as follows:

- PRP prostate injection (to regenerate and rejuvenate healthy tissue in my prostate affected by long standing inflammation).
- PRP penis injection (to regenerate and rejuvenate healthy tissue in my penis affected by long standing inflammation).
- Intraprostatic injection (an injection of antibiotics into my prostate to help kill the remaining staphylococcus aureus bacteria present).
- Fibrinolytic agent (an injection of a special agent to help disintegrate hard tissue that had built up in my penis and prostate).

By 5.15 pm I was free to leave the hospital and get some food. I was really hungry, given I had not eaten since my very light breakfast some ten hours ago.

After a very late lunch I was back to The Central Clinic of Athens at 7 pm to start my second round of intravenous antibiotics for the day. After two-and-a-half hours, at 9.30 pm I took a break from the antibiotics after the first three bottles in order to visit the doctor for a quick prostate PiezoWave.

It was then back to the intravenous clinic to finish my last slowly dripping bottle of Zetalid between 10 and 11.45 pm.

My massive day of prostate injection nine was finally over!

## Friday 19 May

I had my morning intravenous antibiotics between 9.30 am and 1.15 pm. My vein was starting to tire by now so the fluids were taking much longer than normal to drip into me.

The Zetalid was giving me a bit of a stomach ache and I was very tired when I visited the doctor at 1.30 pm.

I had a penis erection PiezoWave and jokingly said to the doctor in advance that I probably only had the energy to give half an erection today. As usual the doctor's pump machine worked its magic and I managed to perform. I also had a prostate PiezoWave – I was close to falling asleep during it. (I was unable to do a prostate massage following yesterday's prostate injection as my prostate was still sensitive.)

The doctor suggested I go to my apartment to eat and rest for the afternoon as the strong antibiotics were starting to take their effect.

After a good afternoon's rest, I was back on the intravenous antibiotics from 6.45 pm to 8.15 pm. The doctor then messaged me to go and have a prostate PiezoWave.

I then finished my last remaining half bottle of Zetalid between 9 pm and 9.30 pm. While undergoing IV antibiotics I spoke to fellow patient George from Germany, whose story you can read at the back of this book. Like me, Chronic Prostatitis really affected George's working life.

## Saturday 20 May

I was back on the intravenous antibiotics between 8.30 am and noon. Following these I went to the doctor to do a quick ten-minute prostate PiezoWave.

After some food and a siesta in the afternoon I was back at the doctor's clinic at 6.45 pm for another prostate PiezoWave. I then went to The Central Clinic of Athens to finish my final batch of antibiotics for the week between 7.30 and 10.30 pm.

I'd done it – I'd made it through prostate injection week nine.

*The entrance to The Central Clinic of Athens where my intravenous antibiotics were administered and where my prostate injections were completed.*

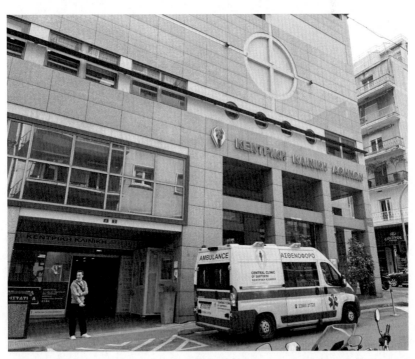

## WEEK 33: Post-prostate injection massaging and monitoring.

### Monday 22 May

During my noon appointment with the doctor I mentioned that I had ejaculated during my sleep last night. I was somewhat concerned this would have flushed out last week's injected antibiotics too early. The doctor said this was fine as the antibiotics were in my prostate for at least three-and-a-half days since last Thursday's prostate injection.

I had a prostate massage which was followed up with a penis erection PiezoWave and prostate PiezoWave.

I explained to the doctor I was still feeling very tired from last week's antibiotics and he said this was perfectly normal. He assured me I would be feeling much stronger in two days.

In the evening at 8.30 I had a prostate massage where the doctor focused on pressing on the area where my last remaining inflammation was. I also had a prostate PiezoWave.

I was hoping that tomorrow, if I had a good night's sleep, that the intravenous antibiotics from last week would be fully worn off.

### Tuesday 23 May

When I awoke this morning, I was feeling much more alert and stronger. Obviously, the antibiotics from last week were exiting my system.

I had a 12.30 pm prostate massage, penis erection PiezoWave and prostate PiezoWave at the doctor's clinic. By now my prostate and urethra seemed to have no sensitive area when pressed, which indicated to me little to no inflammation was left.

In the evening at 7.30 I had another prostate massage and prostate PiezoWave.

## Wednesday 24 May

At 12.30 pm I had a strong prostate massage at the doctor's Central Athens clinic, followed by a penis erection PiezoWave and prostate PiezoWave.

I explained to the doctor how I was still being super diligent with my diet and even threw away a healthy avocado salad yesterday because it had a sweet sauce with some sugar on it.

In the evening at 9.15 I was back at the doctor's clinic having some banter with fellow patient John and Pavlos's wife Elena.

I had a prostate massage, which I immediately followed up with going to urinate. After every prostate massage now, I was trying to immediately get rid of any microbes that may have been pushed out of my prostate and into my urethra during the massage.

I also had a prostate PiezoWave for ten minutes.

## Thursday 25 May

Given it was surgery day for the doctor today I visited the clinic at 9.30 am for my treatment.

I was now feeling much stronger after last week's demanding intravenous antibiotics and prostate injection. I had a very strong prostate massage, penis erection PiezoWave and prostate PiezoWave before heading out for my morning coffee.

In the evening I had a prostate massage and prostate PiezoWave at 9 pm.

## Friday 26 May

At 12.30 pm I received a very strong prostate massage from the doctor. I then completed a penis erection PiezoWave and prostate PiezoWave.

After a great afternoon's rest, I was back at the doctor's clinic at 8.30 pm to do another prostate massage and a prostate PiezoWave.

I said to the doctor's wife, Elena, I was really hoping the treatment would end soon. The constant daily treatment was becoming a mental and physical grind.

## Saturday 27 May

I visited the doctor at 11.45 am to do my familiar prostate massage. The massage was extremely strong and I joked with the doctor whether he'd had spinach for breakfast.

I then had a penis erection PiezoWave and prostate PiezoWave.

I then had a great lunch to catch up with fellow patients Nikos, Christos and George, which was a nice break from the treatment rinse and repeat daily routine.

In the evening at 7 pm I had a prostate massage and prostate PiezoWave to finish my week's treatment.

## WEEK 34: Further prostate massaging and monitoring.

### Monday 29 May

My week started at noon with my now very strong prostate massage, which was followed by a penis erection PiezoWave. I was almost getting used to the daily routine of being given a pump-generated erection then having PiezoWaves shot through my penis to stimulate blood flow and healthy tissue.

I then had a prostate PiezoWave to finish my morning treatment.

After a low-carbohydrate traditional roast pork and Greek salad lunch followed by a siesta, I was back at the doctor's clinic at 8.30 pm. I had a prostate massage and prostate PiezoWave.

I explained to the doctor how I did not feel any nerve tingling or sensation during the prostate PiezoWave. He said this was a good thing as it showed there was limited to no sclerotic tissue left inside my prostate.

## Tuesday 30 May

After a morning coffee with fellow patient Christos, I had a 12.30 pm prostate massage, penis erection PiezoWave and prostate PiezoWave.

The doctor, who does not dish out compliments easily, said I was looking much younger. Given I had now been on a sugar-free, low-carbohydrate, no-alcohol diet for over eight months I was sure my complete prostate and body rejuvenation were progressing extremely well. The effects visually in how I looked were also starting to be commented on by many people.

In the evening the doctor's clinic was really busy with other Chronic Prostatitis sufferers, and I had my prostate massage and prostate PiezoWave at 10.45 pm to round out the day.

## Wednesday 31 May

I had a 12.30 pm prostate massage, penis erection PiezoWave and prostate PiezoWave.

The doctor's secretary, Eugenia, said to me today she was confident that after my injection next week I would be fully cured. After seeing so many patients treated over the years, she was confident I was on the final steps. I hoped and indeed prayed so!

In the evening during my 8.45 pm appointment with the doctor we spoke about all the symptoms that come with Chronic Prostatitis. He explained over the years he had witnessed patients with many strange side effects, including migraines, lower back pain, pelvic pain and neck pain, all of which are a result of a disease in the prostate. I told him to add my blocked ears and extreme lethargy to the symptoms list.

We discussed how Chronic Prostatitis will become big global news over the next five years, due to the simple fact so many men have now had bacteria present in their prostate for several years due to unprotected sexual intercourse or contamination through activities such as swimming in infected swimming pools. Many of these infected males will suffer from enlarged prostates due to Chronic Prostatitis over the coming decade, causing more people to seek medical help.

I had my prostate massage and prostate PiezoWave and was then free to rest.

## Thursday 1 June

I had a noon prostate massage, penis erection PiezoWave and prostate PiezoWave.

It was the same program in the evening at 8.30 pm, but without the penis erection PiezoWave. I just did a prostate massage and prostate PiezoWave.

## Friday 2 June

I had a prostate massage, penis erection PiezoWave (which always starts with a relatively painless intra cavernous injection to send blood to the penile area to support erection) and a prostate PiezoWave at 11.45 am.

I asked the doctor if after next week's injection all would be finished and clear. The doctor said he wanted me to stay until the end of the month to tidy up some things, which was a surprise to me.

I thought I would be free to leave Greece the week after my next injection. I was starting to get very frustrated with how the program kept extending and extending.

In the evening at 8 pm I had a prostate massage and prostate PiezoWave. I was feeling a bit down tonight due to my stay in Athens being extended, yet again. Psychologically it was a real blow having a fixed date you expect to leave but having it change when you are getting so close to it.

### Saturday 3 June

At 10 am I had a prostate massage, penis erection PiezoWave and prostate PiezoWave. I then headed off down the coast to Voula for the weekend to relax prior to injection week ten.

## WEEK 35: Prostate injection ten and another week of intravenous antibiotics.

### Monday 5 June

I was back in Central Athens at the doctor's clinic by 11 am to do my regular prostate massage and PiezoWave treatments.

While waiting I met Erald from Albania, who told me he had completed twenty-one prostate injections. To say I was shocked would be an understatement. I was looking forward to hearing his story over the coming days.

In the evening at 8 pm I had a prostate massage and prostate PiezoWave.

### Tuesday 6 June

I arrived at The Central Clinic of Athens at 8.45 am for my COVID-19 rapid test. After getting the all clear, I went up to the fifth floor to start my intravenous antibiotics in therapy room 502.

The antibiotics started dripping into me at 9.15 am. By 11 am I had taken 250 ml of Voncon, 100 ml of Meronem and 300 ml of Zyxoxid. I then went for a late breakfast before having a prostate massage, penis erection PiezoWave and prostate PiezoWave at the doctor's clinic. By now the antibiotics were starting to kick in and I was feeling a bit lethargic with a stiff neck, so I went to my apartment to rest for the afternoon.

I started my intravenous antibiotics again at 7.30 pm. First, I took the Meronem, followed by the Voncon and then the Zetalid. I finished the three bottles in two hours.

At 9.45 pm I had a prostate massage and prostate PiezoWave to round out the day.

## Wednesday 7 June

I started my intravenous antibiotics at 8 am in The Central Clinic of Athens, stopping half way through my third and final bottle to go visit the doctor to do a uroflow test.

*My twenty-fourth uroflow test showed a maximum urine flow over 30 ml/per second again. This time I registered 32.3 ml/per second which the doctor said was good.*

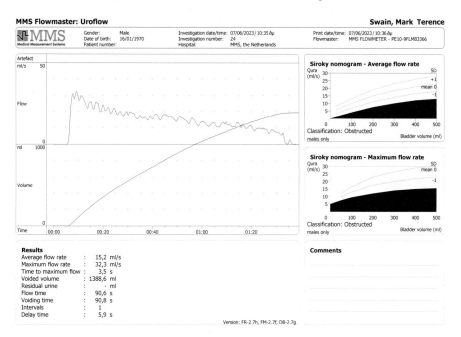

After my uroflow test I went back to The Central Clinic of Athens to finish my remaining half bottle of Zetalid antibiotics. Once my morning antibiotics were finished, I went back to the doctor to do a transrectal prostate scan.

*My fourteenth prostate scan showed a prostate that was*
*8.74 ml in size. It had one very small red inflammation dot*
*right in the centre where the urethra met the prostate.*

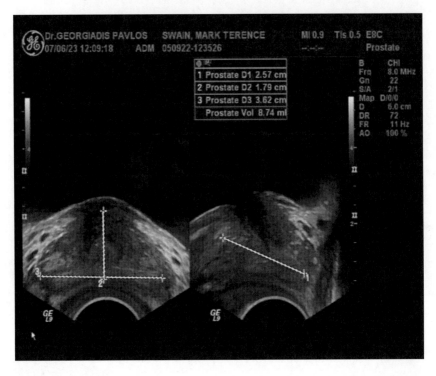

The doctor said tomorrow's injection would eradicate this remaining small piece of inflammation.

Following my prostate scan I had a prostate massage, penis erection PiezoWave and prostate PiezoWave.

After some afternoon rest I started my evening antibiotics at 7 pm with the Meronem first, followed by the Voncon and then the Zetalid. After two-and-a-half hours I was finished and headed to the doctor's clinic at 9.30 pm for a prostate massage and prostate PiezoWave.

## Thursday 8 June

Today was surgery day. First up I visited the doctor at 8 am to do my usual prostate massage, penis erection PiezoWave and prostate

PiezoWave. I then went straight to The Central Clinic of Athens to start my intravenous antibiotics at 9 am.

By 12.15 pm three bottles of antibiotics had dripped into me. I then stayed in the clinic's intravenous treatment ward to await the call down for surgery. At 2 pm a senior nurse came to collect me from my room and I walked with him down to the operating theatre.

*Hooked up to anaesthetic just before my tenth prostate injection.*

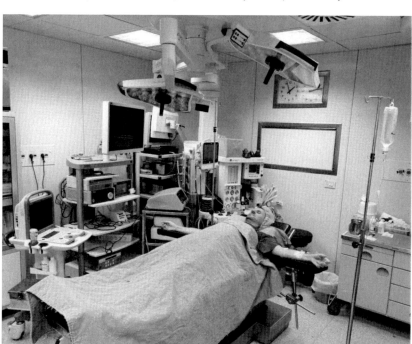

By 3 pm the surgery was complete and I was taken back to the intravenous ward to recover. By 4 pm I felt clear-headed enough to leave the clinic and get some food – I had not eaten since a very small surgery-day breakfast of fruit and nuts.

I rested between 4 and 7 pm before I was back in The Central Clinic of Athens on intravenous antibiotics again at 7.30. I actually started my antibiotics at 8.30 pm and finished them at 10.45 pm.

I then went to the doctor at 11.15 pm for a prostate PiezoWave to finish my big surgery day.

## Friday 9 June

I was back on intravenous antibiotics at 9.15 am to start my fourth and penultimate day of antibiotics for the week. By 11.45 am I had taken on board all three bottles.

I then went straight to the doctor for a penis erection PiezoWave and prostate PiezoWave. After a good afternoon's rest, I was back on intravenous antibiotics at 7.15 pm. The antibiotics were all finished by 9.30 pm.

At 10.15 pm I then did just a prostate PiezoWave given my prostate could not be massaged straight after yesterday's injection.

## Saturday 10 June

I was back in The Central Clinic of Athens on intravenous antibiotics at 8.45 am. Today I started with 100 ml of Meronem, followed by 250 ml of Voncon and then 300 ml of Zyvoxid. After three hours my morning antibiotics were finished.

At noon I visited the doctor to do a penis erection PiezoWave and prostate PiezoWave.

I then had some afternoon rest between 1.30 pm and 6 pm. At 6.30 I went to the doctor to do a quick five-minute prostate PiezoWave. It was then to The Central Clinic of Athens to start my very last round of antibiotics for the week at 6.50 pm.

The three bottles of antibiotics dripped into me really quickly, which was a surprise given I had been using the same vein all week. I was finished by 8 pm and was happy to have the cannula needle taken out of my arm.

I was free to go home and shower without a bandage around my arm and watch the Champions League Final.

I'd done it. I had made it through injection week ten, which would turn out to be my last.

## WEEK 36: Back to prostate massages and monitoring.

### Monday 12 June

At noon I visited the doctor to do my morning program, comprising:

- prostate massage (to smooth out any remaining hard sclerotic tissue in my prostate)
- penis erection PiezoWave (to stimulate the cavernous tissue in my penis and increase blood flow for healing)
- prostate PiezoWave (to break down any long-standing fibrotic tissue or oedemas).

I found the massage quite painful on my sensitive prostate, which had been injected last week. For the first time in a very long time I had to grit my teeth while receiving a prostate massage. This gritting of my teeth would continue during my prostate massages over the next two days.

My complete treatment took around forty minutes before I could leave to stock up with food. I was determined to recharge my body quickly with healthy food following last week's intravenous antibiotics.

I rested a lot in the afternoon as I still felt pretty tired and jaded from last week's gruelling schedule.

In the evening at 9 pm I had a prostate massage and prostate PiezoWave.

### Tuesday 13 June

I advised the doctor I was still feeling pretty lethargic from last week's antibiotics. He suggested I take some high-strength Intelecta

Levocarnitine after my treatment to help my immune system and muscles recover.

*Intelecta Levocarnitine 2g helped me recover from muscle aches and lethargy after a week of intravenous antibiotics.*

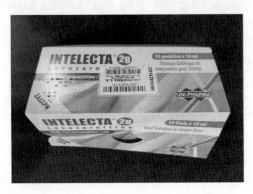

Following our chat I had a prostate massage, penis erection PiezoWave and prostate PiezoWave.

In the evening at 9 pm I had a prostate massage. My prostate still felt very sensitive so the doctor gave me some Voltaren suppositories to insert in my backside overnight to help the inflammation and subdue the mild pain.

I also did a pretty easy prostate PiezoWave for ten minutes.

*The Voltaren suppository to help ease my inflamed prostate following my tenth prostate injection.*

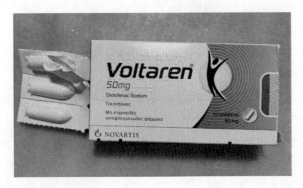

I was looking forward to a good sleep tonight and waking up with more energy.

## Wednesday 14 June

At 1 pm I visited the doctor to have my prostate massage, penis erection PiezoWave and prostate PiezoWave. I was feeling more energetic today, but not yet up to full strength following all the antibiotics I took last week.

In the afternoon I ate some nice steak from the local butcher with fresh market vegetables, and then took a siesta. This was followed by my first afternoon park stroll in a few days. In the evening at 9 pm I visited the doctor to have a prostate massage and prostate PiezoWave.

## Thursday 15 June

I awoke with my now all-too-familiar strong erection. At 11.30 am I visited the doctor and explained my erections were now every night and morning, as well as stronger than ever.

The doctor explained this was the sign of a very healthy urogenital system, particularly the prostate gland. He even said males with a healthy urogenital system should be getting morning erections up to the age of 70 to 75 years old. I hoped I was one of these!

After our discussion I had my regular prostate massage, penis erection PiezoWave and prostate PiezoWave over the course of forty minutes.

I also mentioned to the doctor this morning that my left flank was a bit painful and aching this morning. The doctor said this was the contraction of my iliopsoas muscle, which interestingly was the location of one of my original symptoms.

In the evening I had a prostate massage and prostate PiezoWave. When I arrived back at my apartment my left testicle was aching a bit; again this was like one of my original symptoms.

I was feeling like today my original symptoms were presenting themselves again, but this time they were unravelling.

It was like the nerves and bodily sensation were correcting and going back to what they used to be.

### Friday 16 June

At noon I visited the doctor to have a prostate massage and PiezoWave treatments.

The doctor asked if I would have enough energy to start intravenous antibiotics again next Monday or Tuesday. He wanted to make 100% sure there were no bacteria left at all in my prostate. I said I should be fine to start next Monday as my energy was coming back now following last week's antibiotics. I felt with some further rest and good food over the coming days I would be fine to recommence intravenous antibiotics next week

After my treatment and our discussion, I also stocked up at the nearby pharmacist on my normal daily Norocin and Augmentin antibiotic tablets.

After some rest and good food in the afternoon I had a 9 pm prostate massage and prostate PiezoWave.

### Saturday 17 June

When I visited the doctor this morning, he advised me that the plan for me over the next three weeks was to do three days of intravenous antibiotics each week.

Although my most recent reading of staphylococcus aureus showed a low 3,000 cfu/ml and my most recent prostate scan before my last prostate injection showed very minor inflammation, the doctor said he did not want to leave me with even one microbe.

At noon I proceeded with a prostate massage, penis erection PiezoWave and prostate PiezoWave.

I was back in the clinic again at 7 pm, where I met fellow patient Denis. Denis explained to me how he had similar Chronic Prostatitis symptoms to me, which included back pain, brain swelling and a numb sensation in his leg.

Following our chat, I was called into the doctor's treatment room to have a prostate massage and prostate PiezoWave. Week thirty-six of my treatment was over.

## WEEK 37: Three days of intravenous antibiotics. Prostate PiezoWaves and prostate massages continue.

### Monday 19 June

My week started with a COVID-19 RAT test so I could enter The Central Clinic of Athens. Once I was given the all clear I completed the paperwork to check in for intravenous antibiotics and paid my €300 deposit to start my three days of antibiotic treatment.

I started the IV at 10 am with 100 ml of Meronem dripping into me first, followed by the 250 ml of Voncon and 300 ml of Zyvoxid.

After two-and-a-half hours the three bottles of antibiotics had all dripped into me. I then went to the doctor to have a prostate massage, penis erection PiezoWave and prostate PiezoWave.

While I was waiting to go into the doctor's treatment room, I started chatting with fellow patient Erald. Erald showed me his original prostate scan. I had never seen such an inflamed prostate, and was keen to hear more about his symptoms and journey.

After some rest in the afternoon, I was back on intravenous antibiotics at 7 pm. The three bottles had again taken two-and-a-half hours to drip into me.

Because the cannula was in place just above my left hand near the wrist, I had it taken off after today's treatment as I knew I would not sleep with it in. Every time I bent my left wrist, I felt some mild pain.

Following the IV I went to the doctor at 11 pm for a prostate massage and prostate PiezoWave.

### Tuesday 20 June

My intravenous antibiotics started at 9.15 am. I had another needle put in my right arm, which caused me to sweat profusely as the nurse found the right point to connect the cannula.

I said to myself I only had two days of the cannula in this position and it would soon be over. Once connected to the antibiotics, the three bottles of Meronem, Voncon and Zyvoxid dripped into me over the next hour and a half.

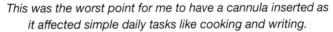

I always found that a fresh vein could take the antibiotics on board so much quicker.

*This was the worst point for me to have a cannula inserted as it affected simple daily tasks like cooking and writing.*

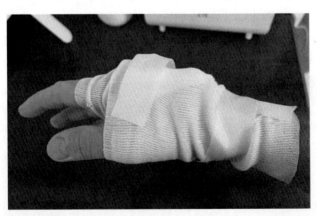

Once I had taken the antibiotics on board, I went to my apartment for a late breakfast before visiting the doctor at 1 pm to have a prostate massage, penis erection PiezoWave and prostate PiezoWave.

It was then time for some afternoon rest as the antibiotics were kicking in and making me a bit tired. I was back on them again from 7 pm until 10 pm, before a visit to the doctor for an end-of-day prostate massage and PiezoWave.

## Wednesday 21 June

My intravenous antibiotics started at 9.15 am and went for three hours. While I was taking on board the antibiotics, I talked to fellow patient Erald again, who shared with me a picture of his original prostate scan. It was probably the worst I had ever seen. (You can read Erald's story at the back of this book.)

I then took a brief food break before visiting the doctor at 2.30 pm for a prostate massage, penis erection PiezoWave and prostate PiezoWave.

*The following two images are of fellow patient Erald's original prostate scan. He had some of the worst prostate inflammation I had ever seen after contracting Chronic Prostatitis from a public swimming pool at around seventeen years of age.*

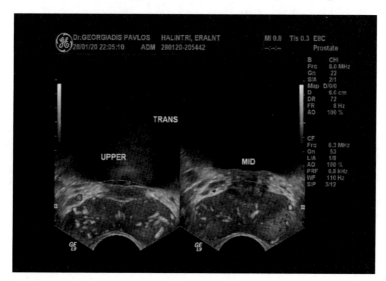

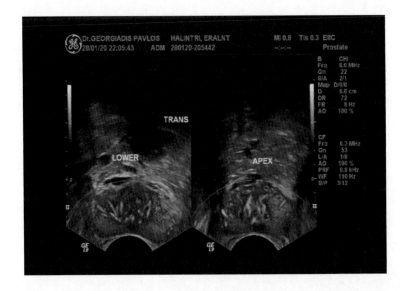

After some rest in the afternoon, I was back in The Central Clinic of Athens taking on board intravenous antibiotics from 7 to 9 pm. This was followed by a 10 pm prostate massage and prostate PiezoWave.

## Thursday 22 June

It was nice to be off the intravenous antibiotics today, especially waking up without a cannula in my arm.

I visited the doctor at 12.30 pm to have a prostate massage, penis erection PiezoWave and prostate PiezoWave. The doctor said to me he would do another transrectal scan on my prostate next Monday after my rest day on Sunday.

At 10 pm I had another prostate massage and prostate PiezoWave.

## Friday 23 June

I woke up with a very strong erection which I seemed to have had for at least an hour. This was becoming a normal start to the day.

Another thing I had noticed was how my ears seemed so much more open and clearer. The doctor later explained that the sexual connection between the prostate and central lobe in the brain was now so much stronger.

## The doctor joked that my sexual capacity was now similar to a healthy twenty-five-year-old male.

Previously when this critical link was cut off by my unhealthy hardened prostate, my ears would block, particularly the right one, and my sexual interest was low.

At noon I had my normal prostate massage and PiezoWave.

In the afternoon I rested away from the 33°C scorching Athens heat, before having an evening prostate massage and prostate PiezoWave at 8.30 pm.

### Saturday 24 June

I visited the doctor for a 11.30 am prostate massage, penis erection PiezoWave and prostate PiezoWave. He asked me if I was feeling good and I replied that I was. My brain felt alert and my energy was high. This was a massive difference to a year ago when I always felt tired and lethargic even after a good night's sleep.

After an afternoon of rest, I had a 6 pm prostate massage and PiezoWave. The doctor and I talked again about how a no-sugar, no-alcohol and low-carbohydrate diet is crucial for a healthy body.

Another week of my treatment was now complete and I was interested to see what my planned prostate scan would show on Monday.

## WEEK 38: Three more days of intravenous antibiotics and continued prostate treatment.

### Monday 26 June

I was at The Central Clinic of Athens at 9.30 am to do my COVID-19 test.

I started the antibiotics at 10.15 am and let the three antibiotic bottles of Meronem, Voncon and Zyvoxid drip into me. I also had, for the first time, some Evaton multivitamins dripped into my right arm, to strengthen my body following all the treatment I'd been having.

By 12.30 pm the fluids were in my veins and I went to the doctor's clinic to do a uroflow test. Following the uroflow test I had a prostate massage, penis erection, PiezoWave and prostate massage. During the prostate PiezoWave, I told the doctor the electromagnetic signals were causing more sensitivity and tingling in my prostate. The doctor said this was good and a sign of healthy tissue.

I then went to my apartment to rest before my next batch of IV started. My intravenous antibiotics commenced again at 7.30 pm and were finished by 9.30 pm.

I then walked the short five-minute walk to the doctor's clinic to do a 10.15 pm prostate massage and prostate PiezoWave.

*The doctor was happy with my twenty-fifth uroflow test, which was much smoother, indicating less strain on my bladder and urethra during urination.*

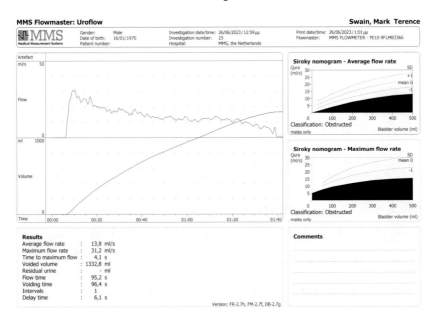

## Tuesday 27 June

I started my intravenous antibiotics at 9 am. Three hours later the three bottles of antibiotics and one bottle of Evaton multivitamins had slowly dripped into my right arm.

While having treatment I felt sorry for fellow patient Alexander in the bed alongside me, who was struggling to have a good vein found by a nurse in which to inject the antibiotics. I could really relate to this horrible situation.

At 1.30 pm I visited the doctor in his clinic for a prostate massage, penis erection PiezoWave and prostate PiezoWave.

I was back on the intravenous antibiotics between 7 and 10 pm. Following this I visited the doctor for an end-of-the-day prostate massage and prostate PiezoWave.

## Wednesday 28 June

I was back on the intravenous antibiotics in The Central Clinic of Athens at 9 am. The three bottles of antibiotics and one bottle of multivitamins dripped into my right arm over two hours.

After a late breakfast I was back in the doctor's clinic at 12.30 pm to do my normal morning prostate massage and PiezoWave treatment.

From 7 pm to 8.15 pm I took on board my last three bottles of antibiotics for the week. It was so good to have the cannula disconnected, knowing my next shower would be without restriction.

I then visited the doctor at 8.30 pm to do my end-of-day prostate massage and PiezoWave.

## Thursday 29 June

I visited the doctor at 1 pm to do an assessment transrectal scan of my prostate. This would be a very important scan for me given I was due to be near the end of my treatment.

The doctor said it was difficult to know if this inflammation was just a residual inflammation. After careful consideration he said I should go to the microbiological laboratory tomorrow to do a sperm examination. He particularly wanted to get a read on my leukocyte white blood cell count to determine if my body was still fighting any form of infection or bacteria. Any number below two on the leukocyte scale would be a good sign.

The doctor also decided to start me on a new oral antibiotic immediately called Vibramycin, in an effort to fight any staphylococcus aureus that may be remaining.

*My fifteenth prostate scan still showed some mild inflammation. The prostate had reduced in size by 0.02 ml to 8.72 ml.*

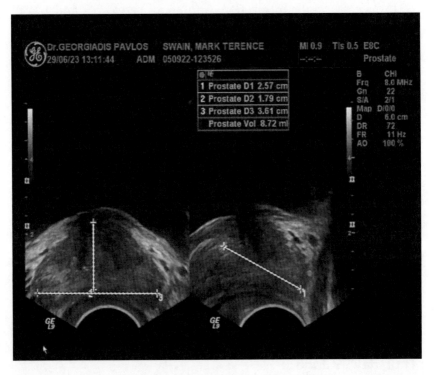

Following the transrectal scan I had a prostate massage, penis erection PiezoWave and prostate PiezoWave. At 10 pm I had a prostate massage and prostate PiezoWave.

## Friday 30 June

I had an earlier appointment with the doctor today as he wanted to send me to the microbiological laboratory to get an updated sperm test. He was particularly keen to get my white blood cell reading.

At 9.30 am I had a penis erection PiezoWave and prostate PiezoWave. I urinated afterwards at the request of the doctor as he then wanted to perform a prostate massage on me. The goal of this prostate massage was to ensure my sperm would give the most accurate biological reading when I went to the Mycolab laboratory.

After the doctor's treatment I took a taxi to Mycolab. I duly hit the reclining chair in the patient room and deposited another sperm sample in the plastic tube the receptionist gave me. She said I would have the leukocyte reading on my sperm sample by midday the same day.

I visited the doctor again at 8.30 pm and he explained he was surprised the leukocytes in my white blood cell test were as high as they were. He wanted me to ejaculate tomorrow and then do another sperm test next Tuesday. Based on the reading of this new sperm leukocyte test he would determine if I needed to do another prostate injection next week.

Given the bad news of the high leukocyte reading I felt surprisingly upbeat. I think it was because I was reading the book *On Fire* by John O'Leary, which is about a nine-year-old boy who had to recover from severe burns over ninety percent of his body.

My attitude was, at least I was feeling great and in good hands with the doctor.

*The leukocyte sperm test indeed came back right on time and
showed a reading of a few white blood cells (10–12) per field.*

---

Ιδιωτικό Διαγνωστικό Εργαστήριο Ειδικών Λοιμώξεων - Μυκητιάσεων & Μικροβιολογικών Εξετάσεων
• Τμήμα Βιοπαθολογίας (Ορμονολογικό-Βιοχημικό-Αιματολογικό-Ανοσολογικό) - Μοριακής Βιολογίας - Προγεννητικού Ελέγχου
• Τμήμα Κυτταρολογίας - Εργαστήριο Ψηφιακής Ανάλυσης Εικόνας
(Digital Image Analysis Lab)

Λεωφ. Κηφισίας, 354 Χαλάνδρι Τ.Κ. 15233
ΑΦΜ:998012799 - ΔΟΥ: ΧΑΛΑΝΔΡΙΟΥ
Τηλ. 210-8028817, 210-6890505 Φαξ: 210-6890506
www.mycolab.gr - info@mycolab.gr

Patient name:     MARK SWAIN                              DATE:     30/06/2023

### CULTURE  OF SPERM

Leukocytes (White Blood Cells):     Few (10-12) per fied
Stem Fungus:
Neisser:
Gramm stain:

**Cultivation (aerobic)**

**Cultivation (anaerobic)**

**Chamydiaceae:**

**Mycoplasma Fermentans**

**Mycoplasma Hominis:**

**Ureaplasma Urealyticum:**

   **COMMENTS**

### Saturday 1 July

I visited the doctor at 11.30 am to do my prostate massage, penis erection PiezoWave and prostate PiezoWave.

The doctor and I discussed my high leukocyte results again and agreed I would do another sperm test next week. The doctor said if my leukocytes were less than five, we would not do a prostate injection next week. If the leukocytes were higher than five, we would.

At 6 pm I had a prostate massage and prostate PiezoWave to finish another emotional rollercoaster of a week.

## WEEK 39: Four days of intravenous antibiotics. No prostate injection.

### Monday 3 July

I visited the doctor at 11.45 am to start the week with my prostate massage and PiezoWave treatments.

Because the microbiologist was away tomorrow, I would do my planned sperm leukocyte test this coming Wednesday instead. This test would be pivotal in determining my next treatment steps.

At 9 pm I had a prostate massage and prostate PiezoWave.

The doctor was taking some vacation leave next week, so I only had five more days to get through this week before a much-needed break.

### Tuesday 4 July

I was back in the doctor's clinic at 11.30 am for my 11.45 am appointment.

While waiting I took another very close look at my last prostate scan and noticed a very small red dot, which I mentioned to the doctor.

*Upon reviewing one of my last prostate scan images again
I noticed a small red dot on the mid left side.*

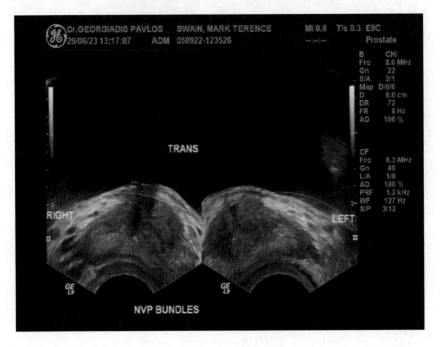

The doctor said I would start intravenous antibiotics tomorrow and he would decide if I had another prostate injection done once he had reviewed the new sperm test results. I proceeded after our discussions to have a prostate massage, penis erection PiezoWave and prostate PiezoWave.

At 8.30 pm I had a prostate massage and prostate PiezoWave. When I was leaving the doctor's clinic I bumped into a fellow patient, who I did not know by name yet. What I did know, though, was I was stunned regarding how much younger he was looking compared to when I first saw him a month or so ago.

## Wednesday 5 July

Today was going to be a busy day.

I started off in the doctor's clinic at 8 am with a penis erection PiezoWave, prostate PiezoWave and lastly a heavy prostate massage. I was then sent to the Mycolab microbiological test centre to do a leukocyte white blood cell test of my sperm. I was then back to The Central Clinic of Athens to start intravenous antibiotics.

The nurse struggled to find a good vein in my now peppered arms. I sweated profusely as she tried a couple of points, but despite injecting and swirling the needle she was unable to get a good connection.

I was very close to saying stop, I can take no more of this.

Finally, she found a vein in my right forearm. I could start taking on board my 200 ml of Voncon, 250 ml of Meronem and 300 ml of Zyvoxid.

After two bottles of antibiotics the Mycolab sperm test result popped up on my phone. My leukocytes had reduced from few (10–12) per field to rare (3–4) per field over the last five days.

The doctor however said my bladder was too full, at nearly 1.4 litres. This was causing some of the volatility of flow you see above as I was straining to get a large amount of urine out of my bladder.

Following the uroflow I went back to The Central Clinic of Athens to finish my last bottle of antibiotics. It was now 3 pm and time for a very late breakfast and afternoon nap.

At 8 pm I was back on intravenous antibiotics again. I had one bottle before stopping for a while to visit the doctor for a prostate massage and prostate PiezoWave. I then returned to the Clinic between 10 pm and 12.35 am to finish the last two bottles of Meronem and Zyvoxid.

A long, demanding day was over!

*My leukocytes had reduced from few (10–12) per field to rare
(3–4) per field over the last five days.*

---

**Ιδιωτικό Διαγνωστικό Εργαστήριο Ειδικών Λοιμώξεων – Μυκητιάσεων & Μικροβιολογικών Εξετάσεων**
• **Τμήμα Βιοπαθολογίας** (Ορμονολογικό-Βιοχημικό-Αιματολογικό-Ανοσολογικό) – **Μοριακής Βιολογίας - Προγεννητικού Ελέγχου**
• **Τμήμα Κυτταρολογίας - Εργαστήριο Ψηφιακής Ανάλυσης Εικόνας**
**(Digital Image Analysis Lab)**

Λεωφ. Κηφισίας, 354 Χαλάνδρι Τ.Κ. 15233
ΑΦΜ:998012799 - ΔΟΥ: ΧΑΛΑΝΔΡΙΟΥ
Τηλ. 210-8028817, 210-6890505 Φαξ: 210-6890506
www.mycolab.gr - info@mycolab.gr

| Patient name: | MARK SWAIN | DATE: | 05/07/2023 |
|---|---|---|---|

**CULTURE OF SPERM**

Leukocytes (White Blood Cells):    Rare ( 3-4) per field
Stem Fungus:
Neisser:
Gramm stain:

**Cultivation (aerobic)**

**Cultivation (anaerobic)**

**Chamydiaceae:**

**Mycoplasma Fermentans**

**Mycoplasma Hominis:**

**Ureaplasma Urealyticum:**

**COMMENTS**

---

I interrupted the antibiotics after two bottles to visit the doctor
and do a uroflow test.

*My latest uroflow test (the twenty-seventh) showed*
*a maximum flow of 31.2 ml/per second.*

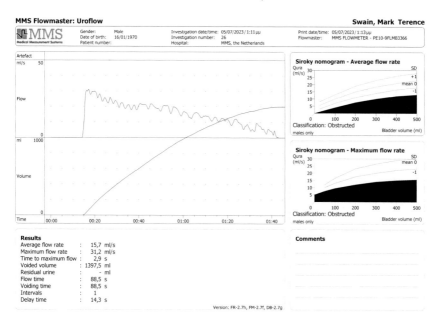

## Thursday 6 July

At 8.30 am I started my intravenous antibiotics again, which took four hours to steadily and slowly drip into me. I then walked the five short minutes from The Central Clinic of Athens to the doctor's clinic at Asklipiou Street, number thirty-nine.

There I had a prostate massage, penis erection PiezoWave and prostate PiezoWave. I felt some penis tingling during the prostate PiezoWave, which indicated some final fibrotic tissue may be breaking down.

The doctor explained to me that in the next sperm test I would do after my upcoming break on 20 July, he was confident my leukocytes would show the desired reading between zero and one, which means no infection.

At 7.30 pm I had a prostate massage and prostate PiezoWave. This was followed by three hours of intravenous antibiotics.

## Friday 7 July

I started my three bottles of antibiotics plus a bottle of Evaton vitamins intravenously at 8.30 am.

The fluids had all slowly dripped into me by 11.30 am. After a late breakfast I went to the doctor at 12.30 pm to do my prostate massage, penis erection PiezoWave and prostate PiezoWave.

**The doctor explained that following my last batch of intravenous antibiotics tomorrow evening, I would stop all antibiotics in readiness for my next planned sperm test on 20 July.**

Stopping all antibiotics for around twelve days gives the most accurate microbiological results. I was really tired from this week's antibiotics as I dragged myself back to The Central Clinic of Athens for another intravenous session that started at 7 pm.

I wearily took on board the first bottle of Voncon, before the doctor messaged me to head up to the clinic. There I had a prostate massage and PiezoWave. It was then back to The Central Clinic for more intravenous antibiotics between 9 and 11.30 pm.

## Saturday 8 July

I started my final day of antibiotics at 8.30 am and finished them at 11.30 am. In total I consumed 200 ml of Voncon, 250 ml of Meronem and 300 ml of Zyvoxid antibiotics. I also took on board 150 ml of Evaton multivitamins. I then had a prostate massage, penis erection PiezoWave and prostate PiezoWave.

At 6 pm I visited the doctor again for my last appointment before my break. I received a very strong prostate massage from him and a prostate PiezoWave.

At 7 pm I was in The Central Clinic of Athens for two bottles of intravenous antibiotics, 200 ml of Voncon and 200 ml of Meronem.

*I was so happy to disconnect my vein after another four days of intravenous antibiotics.*

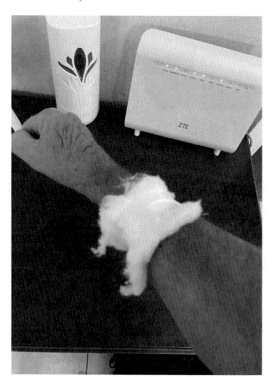

I was now free to go on my vacation.

## Eleven days break. All antibiotics stopped.

This was a break I really needed. It was so good to have eleven days off to tour around the beautiful Peloponnese region of Greece. I had so much more energy than before my treatment to drive daily, go sightseeing, swimming, and generally be a very active tourist.

I had the energy to walk at least six kilometres every day and woke up refreshed after a good night's sleep, something that never happened to me in the past.

One day I caught up with fellow patient Christos who was in the area.

*Drinking my first freddo espresso cold coffee with fellow patient Christos in Monemvasia as the summer temperatures started to rise in Greece.*

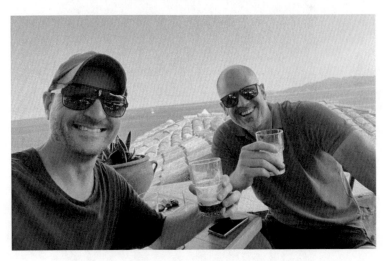

I stuck rigidly to my prescribed diet and stayed completely off the antibiotics during this break, as prescribed by the doctor.

I felt a bundle of energy as I headed back to Athens. I also attended two great concerts from Andrea Bocelli and The Arctic Monkeys before I went back to my treatment again.

I really did feel like my old self again, before I even knew what Chronic Prostatitis was. It felt to me that I really had got my life back.

## My final test and all clear result

### Thursday 20 July

After my antibiotic-free eleven-day break, I was back at the doctor's clinic at 9 am.

I explained to the doctor I felt very healthy and well during my time off. I proceeded to have a penis erection PiezoWave and prostate massage. I certainly had not missed the routine of these daily treatments during my time off! Following my prostate massage, I was sent to the Mycolab laboratory test centre to do another sperm test. I was hoping this would be my last.

I was now free to leave Greece while I awaited my sperm analysis results. This would take around nine days. I departed Athens airport en route to London Luton airport to visit my mother. I had a real spring and positivity in my step.

When I landed and I was waiting to collect my luggage, this however changed. The first phase of my sperm tests results came through showing the white blood cell leukocytes were still three to four per field, when I was expecting them to be zero to one per field.

I decided not to contact the doctor or the Mycolab laboratory regarding these results. I wanted to see what the full microbiological results were when they came through in about a week.

On Wednesday 26 July 2023, a date that I will never forget, my microbiological results came through all clear. I had no bacteria remaining in my prostate.

I immediately messaged the doctor and asked, 'Does this mean I'm microbe free?' His response was:

You are considered cured, since there is a progressive decrease in the number of leukocytes and no bacteria. Although there are 3–4 leukocytes after a month or more, the number will fall to 0–1 or 1–2.

I also called Jiota at Mycolab laboratory to get her opinion. She also said that I was all clear now and would not need any more treatment.

I was absolutely delighted, almost in tears and excited about getting my life back again.

*The white blood cell count on my last sperm test*
*showed a reading of 3–4 per field.*

Ιδιωτικό Διαγνωστικό Εργαστήριο Ειδικών Λοιμώξεων - Μυκητιάσεων & Μικροβιολογικών Εξετάσεων
• Τμήμα Βιοπαθολογίας (Ορμονολογικό-Βιοχημικό-Αιματολογικό-Ανοσολονικό) - Μοριακής Βιολογίας - Προγεννητικού Ελέγχου
• Τμήμα Κυτταρολογίας - Εργαστήριο Ψηφιακής Ανάλυσης Εικόνας
(Digital Image Analysis Lab)

Λεωφ. Κηφισίας 354 Χαλάνδρι Τ.Κ. 15233
ΑΦΜ:998012799 - ΔΟΥ: ΧΑΛΑΝΔΡΙΟΥ
Τηλ. 210-8028817, 210-6890505 Φαξ: 210-6890506
www.mycolab.gr - info@mycolab.gr

| Patient name: | MARK SWAIN | DATE: | 20/07/2023 |

### CULTURE OF SPERM

Leukocytes (White Blood Cells):    Rare (3-4) per field

Stem Fungus:

Neisser:

Gramm stain:


**Cultivation (aerobic)**


**Cultivation (anaerobic)**


**Chamydiaceae:**


**Mycoplasma Fermentans**


**Mycoplasma Hominis:**


**Ureaplasma Urealyticum:**


**COMMENTS**

*My final Mycolab sperm analysis report showing
no microbes were present.*

Ιδιωτικό Διαγνωστικό Εργαστήριο Ειδικών Λοιμώξεων - Μυκητιάσεων & Μικροβιολογικών Εξετάσεων
• Τμήμα Βιοπαθολογίας (Ορμονολογικό-Βιοχημικό-Αιμοτολογικό-Ανοσολογικό) - Μοριακής Βιολογίας - Προγεννητικού Ελέγχου
• Τμήμα Κυτταρολογίας - Εργαστήριο Ψηφιακής Ανάλυσης Εικόνας
(Digital Image Analysis Lab)

Λεωφ. Κηφισίας 354 Χαλάνδρι Τ.Κ. 15233
ΑΦΜ:998012799 - ΔΟΥ: ΧΑΛΑΝΔΡΙΟΥ
Τηλ. 210-8028817, 210-6890505 Fax: 210-6890506
www.mycolab.gr - info@mycolab.gr

Patient name:   MARK SWAIN                                    DATE:       20/07/2023

## CULTURE OF SPERM

Leukocytes (White Blood Cells):   Rare (3-4) per field
Stem Fungus:                      NEGATIVE (-)
Neisser:                          NEGATIVE (-)
Gramm stain:                      NEGATIVE (-)

**Cultivation (aerobic)**
NEGATIVE (-)
**Cultivation (anaerobic)**
NEGATIVE (-)

**Chamydiaceae:**
NEGATIVE (-)

**Mycoplasma Fermentans**
NEGATIVE (-)

**Mycoplasma Hominis:**
NEGATIVE (-)

**Ureaplasma Urealyticum:**
NEGATIVE (-)

**COMMENTS**
Ph 7.8  -  Hb Erythrocytes (0-1) per field

255

## Six month check up

### Tuesday 30th January 2024

I arrived back in a chilly five degrees Athens for a check up six months after my original all clear. I wanted the peace of mind that everything was perfect with my prostate and overall health before launching this book.

It was strange walking the streets I had walked so many times before from Panepistimio metro station to the doctor's office.

On arrival I was happy to see the doctor again and quickly proceeded to do the urine uroflow test and prostate transrectal scan.

*My urine had a decent flow and consistency given the 766.2 ml present in my bladder.*

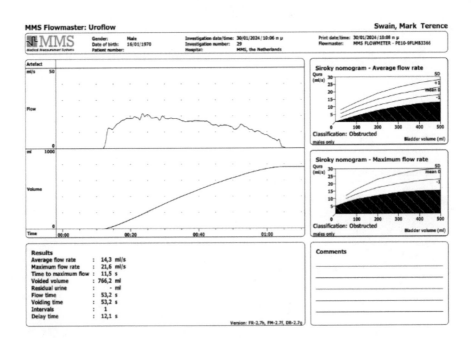

*My first transrectal scan in over six months showed a healthy prostate with no inflammation. My prostate was around the same size as when I left Athens in July 2023 at 8.84ml.*

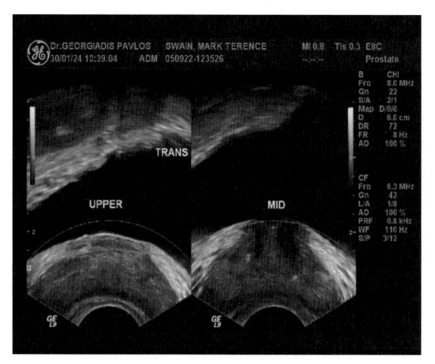

Following my transrectal scan I had a prostate massage, which was not painful at all and caused me no sweating. I then took a taxi to the Mycolab sperm test clinic to leave a deposit for analysis.

A week later when I had arrived back in Australia my results came through. I was delighted to read there was no bacteria present in my prostate and also that my white blood cell count of leukocytes was 0–1.

This reading demonstrated that my body was fighting no infection and was a million miles away from the leukocyte reading of 35–40 I had when I arrived in Athens with Chronic Prostatitis.

*My six-month check up showed a 100% clean bill of health with no bacterial microbes in my prostate and a healthy blood leukocyte reading of 0–1..*

Ιδιωτικό Διαγνωστικό Εργαστήριο Ειδικών Λοιμώξεων - Μυκητιάσεων & Μικροβιολογικών Εξετάσεων
• Τμήμα Βιοπαθολογίας (Ορμονολογικό-Βιοχημικό-Αιματολογικό-Ανοσολογικό) - Μοριακής Βιολογίας - Προγεννητικού Ελέγχου
• Τμήμα Κυτταρολογίας - Εργαστήριο Ψηφιακής Ανάλυσης Εικόνας
(Digital Image Analysis Lab)

**mycolab**

Λεωφ. Κηφισίας 354 Χαλάνδρι Τ.Κ. 15233
ΑρΜ:998012799 - ΔΟΥ: ΧΑΛΑΝΔΡΙΟΥ
Τηλ. 210-8028817, 210-6890505 Φαξ: 210-6890506
www.mycolab.gr - Info@mycolab.gr

Patient name:   MARK SWAIN                    DATE:      30/01/2024

### CULTURE OF SPERM

Leukocytes (White Blood Cells):   Rarely (0-1) per field
Stem Fungus:                      NEGATINE (-)
Neisser:                          NEGATIVE (-)
Gramm stain:                      NEGATIVE (-)

**Cultivation (aerobic)**
NEGATIVE (-)
**Cultivation (anaerobic)**
NEGATIVE (-)

**Chamydiaceae:**
NEGATIVE (-) Molecular analysis

**Mycoplasma Fermentans**
NEGATIVE (-)

**Mycoplasma Hominis:**
NEGATIVE (-)

**Ureaplasma Urealyticum:**
NEGATIVE (-)

**COMMENTS**
PH 7.8  -  Hb (-) Erythrocytes (0-1) per field

This final reading was a relief to me and demonstrated that my body was no longer fighting the debilitating effects of Chronic Prostatitis.

I had cured Chronic Prostatitis and got my life back.

## Conclusion

During 2020, I felt like I had a serious health problem. I was stunned at how my body was deteriorating and how I was experiencing so many weird symptoms. I spent thousands of dollars visiting various doctors and specialists in Australia with the following main symptoms:

- excruciating lower back pain
- terrible lethargy
- pain in my left flank
- frequent urination
- brain swelling and ears blocking.

Over the course of 2020 and 2021, I visited general practitioners, chiropractors, physiotherapists, gastroenterologists, ear, nose and throat specialists, infectious diseases specialists, urologists, acupuncturists and more.

Every test and every check I had came back with: you are okay.

'You are perfectly healthy,' was the usual response. I even had, 'It's probably just COVID-related stress'.

But I knew something was wrong. I felt like I was slowly dying. I went from feeling forty years old to seventy years old in six months.

As you now know, I went on to trusty Dr Google and started typing in my symptoms to see what came back. A problem with my prostate seemed to be a possibility. You now know the rest of the story.

However, I often think, what if I had not remained so determined to find a solution to my problems? What if I had accepted the specialists' responses that 'you are okay'? The simple fact is I would be in an even worse physical condition, have a poor quality of life, be racked with anxiety and worry, and be on a fast track to prostate cancer.

I have written this book not for sympathy, but to implore all of you out there who are not feeling yourself to get a third, fourth or fifth opinion until you have an answer.

I have created a website www.chronicprostatitis.org, and case studies to help other people suffering from this terrible disease. My hope is if you read the case studies that follow, which are across men from ages ranging from twenty-two years old to sixty years old, you can better identify if you have Chronic Prostatitis symptoms.

With prostate problems affecting up to seven in ten men globally, my hope is if you do have a problem, you can diagnose it early. If I save one person from the agony I went through by creating this website and writing this book, I will be happy.

As for me, after the toughest ten months of my life, I'm happy to say I'm totally healthy again, feeling fitter than ever and delighted that I got my life back.

# PART III
# CASE STUDIES

# 6

# CASE STUDIES OF OTHER PATIENTS

## Christo's story (thirty-nine years old)

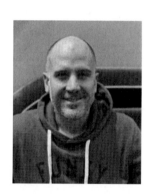

### Summary

In June 2017, Christos noticed he was regularly getting up in the night to urinate; this had never happened to him before.

This lasted for several months, by which time Christos was getting up once or twice every night to pee. In August his mother suggested he get a prostate examination given his age and symptoms. At this stage his prostate was 24 ml and no problems were identified by the doctor who checked him.

By September 2017, things got worse: when Christos urinated the flow would just completely stop in the middle of urination like it had been cut off. He was also experiencing a huge burning feeling in his abdominal area. Christos knew something was wrong.

He would often have a big desire to urinate or defecate but nothing would come out. He also had a fever around this time and a temperature of 38°C.

Christos decided to visit a general doctor and he separately took a urine test to a lab for examination. The doctor said Christos had cystitis and gave a prescription for Augmentin tablets for ten days.

Christos was happy he now knew what the problem was and felt relieved. He started on the medicine, but there was little improvement. His urination result showed that Klebsiella pneumonia was present. Christos called his doctor to advise him of the bacteria discovered in the urination test, and he carried on taking Augmentin for nine days. He was still however getting a huge burning sensation in his perineum.

The next step was for Christos to visit a urologist. Christos told the urologist about the bacteria and his symptoms. The urologist said Christos had acute Prostatitis which would pass, but his tablets needed to be changed to Ciprofloxacin for ten days.

From the first Ciprofloxacin tablet Christos felt almost perfect and he continued to take the remaining tablets over nine more days. Christos felt really good but on the ninth day he ejaculated and it felt like a knife was pushed into his perineum and under his scrotum. The pain Christos was experiencing after ejaculating was tremendous. He went back to the urologist who extended the treatment with thirty days of Glimbax antibiotics.

Every time Christos took the Glimbax tablet he had terrible pain for around five hours in his perineum. Christos went to another doctor who wrote a prescription for a Bricklin antibiotic which was injected into his backside twice a day for six days. This medicine provided very good pain relief. Christos also kept on the Glimbax tablets and was only experiencing minor pain.

As soon as Christos stopped these injections and tablets, a very strong nerve pain and strong burning came back to his perineum. Christos decided to go to the hospital for checks on his abdomen, bladder and an ultrasound before and after urination. He also did a urine and sperm test. The doctor said everything was all clear and healthy. By this point Christo's prostate had enlarged to 35 ml in size.

Between November 2017 and January 2018, Christos visited three more urologists. The pain he was experiencing by now was so strong he could not even sleep properly; he would wake every hour with a very strong burning in his perineum.

All the urologists Christos visited around this time said he needed to go on living with these symptoms, and the one who did a prostate finger examination said he had a soft, healthy prostate.

By March 2018 with the pain and anxiety Christos was experiencing he had a panic attack. He started feeling dizzy, he was filled with anger and started crying all day. He wanted to rip out his perineum due to the pain.

Christos said to his girlfriend at this point he cannot go on living like this. His girlfriend recommended Christos see a psychologist and Christos called an SOS doctor who arrived at his house in half an hour. The doctor provided a Xanax anxiety pill which really made him calm down and he felt a little better. The doctor advised Christos he needed to keep on the Xanax tablets and another anti-depressant called Dumyrox to overcome his worry and anger.

Christos started taking the Xanax in March 2018 for a month and the Dumyrox for five months.

In November 2018, Christos had unprotected sex with his girl-friend and he started having symptoms again. His perineum was in strong pain like a foreign body was tingling and pressing him. Christos tried to live without ejaculating given the pain when doing this, and he also kept a healthy diet.

In September 2019, Christos had unprotected sex with his girl-friend again and straight away he had perineum pain with strong burning and pressure; he also felt like his urethra was getting bigger.

Christos went to the doctor again and asked for some relief. He was given Glimbax antibiotics for three weeks and felt less pain.

By March 2020, Christos experienced a new symptom with his abdomen swelling up and becoming painful; he went back to his psychologist to prescribe Xanax and Dumyrox again. Christos stayed on the Dumyrox for nine months.

Christos around this time visited another urologist who prescribed Zithromax and Doxycycline. After these tablets Christos felt really good. His abdomen muscles released and after ejaculation his left flank muscles relaxed. His urination flow was strong, erections were strong and he was largely pain free.

By July 2021, Christos was getting more pain again (this time in his left flank), muscle tightness in his abdomen, lots of internal gas, even stronger perineum pain, a swollen abdomen and now lower back pain. Christos was injected with Briklin again over three days and started taking Levofloxacin for thirty days. The pain had subsided by August but Christos still had left flank and left testicle pain.

By September 2021, the fatigue really started to kick in. Christos was working out at the gym daily and also running but he felt more and more tired. He was also taking Xanax and Ladose antidepressants between September 2021 and February 2022.

In February 2022, Christos started taking Glimbax on his own and started to feel a bit better. However, as soon as he stopped the tablets, he had a huge burning in his prostate area and a feeling of exploding inflammation.

Christos went to a new doctor who did a sperm examination which showed staphylococcus was present. Christos was prescribed Doxycycline, Clarithromycin and Cotrimoxazole for two months. Christos also had PiezoWave treatment on his perineum for five sessions to help the antibiotics go into his prostate.

By July 2022, Christos quit his job because of all the pain, anxiety and uncertainty in his life. He felt really exhausted and wanted to stop work to try to relax from a stressful job and get better.

With symptoms of burning perineum, weight in perineum, swollen abdomen, excess gas, very frequent urination and back pain ever present, Christos visited Dr Pavlos Georgiadis in March 2023.

## Treatment

Christos's fist examination from Dr Pavlos Georgiadis showed a heavily swollen prostate through a transrectal scan. His sperm test showed staphylococcus lugdunensis and morganella morganii bacteria were present.

Christos started prostate massages daily and he felt a lift and pain relief after the first massage. His urination was also much stronger. After a few weeks of treatment his sleeping became much better and he did not need to get up at night to urinate.

Christos has more treatment ahead of him but he can now see light at the end of the tunnel and is on a path to getting his life back.

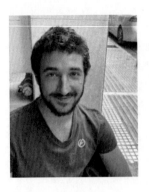

## Dimos's story (twenty-two years old)

### Summary

In July 2019, Dimos had sex with a female during a one-night stand and the condom broke. This caused Dimos to go for a sperm test at his local doctor. This initial sperm test showed staphylococcus was present. Ceclor antibiotics were taken for ten days.

A follow-up sperm test was negative for microbes and the burning during urination symptoms subsided for a while. A few weeks later after taking Ceclor antibiotics, an annoying sensation (not burning) happened during urination. Dimos also felt as if more urine should flow.

Staphylococcus showed up in a subsequent sperm test and Dimos was advised to have Ufexil antibiotics, and he undertook three antibacterial injections in the urethra.

Over a period of a year-and-a-half Dimos had seven visits to one doctor alone, to be told:

## I can't find anything wrong with you.

After leaving things for a year-and-a-half and believing he was partly crazy, Dimos then started to notice new symptoms of erectile dysfunction and a noticeable burning sensation during and after urination. Dimos also felt like he could not properly clear his bladder, and it felt as if his urination was obstructed.

He started to feel tired regularly even though he was getting enough sleep. All this started to have an impact on his psychological health. Gut issues also started to appear, with more regular gas. Stomach pain was starting to be felt in his lower abdomen.

Only small drops would come out during the last moments of urination when he felt his bladder had more to give.

By December 2021, some two-and-a-half years after the initial sexual encounter, symptoms worsened further with a pulse beating in different parts of his body, including his upper left chest above the heart and on the left thigh.

Dimos felt sixty to seventy years old at this point, despite being only twenty-two. He stopped his university studies and moved to Athens to seek further medical opinion. The stress of stopping his studies and worrying about his symptoms started to cause more pronounced beating in the upper chest.

Dimos undertook another sperm test with a different doctor, who also wanted a prostate fluid test which required a prostate massage first. The result showed a new form of bacteria present, staphylococcus coagulase negative. After this he was prescribed Ciproxin for four weeks and then showed negative again for all microbes.

Dimos also visited a cardiologist in January 2022 because of the pulses in his chest and the fact he constantly felt tired. These problems were worst when he was stressed, which even caused Dimos to think he had a problem in his head.

At this point, and still with symptoms, Dimos visited Dr Pavlos Georgiadis.

## Treatment

Dimos undertook a uroflow test, transrectal scan, bladder scan, testicle scan and ultrasound. He also undertook a sperm test after a rigorous prostate massage. The tests showed inflammation in the prostate. The doctor also demonstrated that there was restriction in the urethra causing obstructed urine flow.

Ten days later the sperm test results came back showing infection with the following microbes:

* staphylococcus aureus

- staphylococcus haemolyticus
- mycoplasma hominis
- ureaplasma urealyticum.

In September 2022, twice-daily prostate massages started. Dimos's stomach pain started immediately reducing and the antibiotics prescribed caused less burning sensation.

The new antibiotics also generated a better uroflow result and some improvement in urethra restriction with better maximum flow rate. As prostate massages became more frequent, Dimos's energy and tiredness improved and there were fewer problems getting erections. These erections were also becoming stronger.

## Current symptoms

Dimos still gets nerve pain in his back and neck. He feels as if there is a weight on his back at times. Dimos still does not fully feel his old self yet despite being only twenty-two years old. He still feels much older than his age. 'I probably feel forty to fifty years old right now,' Dimos freely admitted.

The main reason Dimos sought this treatment program was his inability to have erections and he felt his brain could not function properly. In Dimos's words, 'I had a cloudy mind; it was not sharp. My mind was so easily tired. It felt like some weight and pressure was on my brain.'

'The disease changed my personality one hundred and eighty degrees. I was the type of guy who was not afraid of anything and could face even the most difficult tasks. My mentality used to be, give me problems to fight. This has changed as I have concerns about not feeling that strong and my mind is not that focused on positive things.'

'Before the symptoms, if you cut my hand, I would still feel okay.' Taking male productivity this young is killing him in life.

Dimos's treatment is continuing and he is already feeling healthier and has less prostate inflammation and better urinary flow.

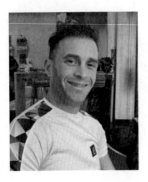

## Vaggelis's story (thirty-four years old)

### Summary

Vaggelis had been peeing too much since he was twenty-one years old. He never really paid it that much attention and got used to it. When he was twenty-seven years old, he had surgery on his nose and the doctor advised him that he had a problem with his liver. The doctor recommended he have it checked out and he went for a general examination.

Vaggelis was told your liver is okay, but you have an infection in your prostate. At this stage Vaggelis didn't pay attention to this as he generally felt fine.

After about a year his peeing became very annoying; it was affecting his appointments at work as he constantly felt he needed to urinate. It was difficult having regular and urgent urination when he was hosting property viewings. He also could not sleep properly at night and was waking every two to three hours to get up and pee.

He decided to visit a doctor again, who did an examination and prescribed Glimbax tablets for a month. He took the pills but started having very strong pain in his prostate. It was hurting so much he could not even sit on his motorcycle. The doctor told him to be patient and complete the month of tablets.

Two weeks after completing the tablets he started to notice problems having erections. At this stage he went to another doctor who advised him prostatitis was not important or linked to erectile dysfunction. The doctor recommended he have a doppler examination to check the blood vessels in his penis. Vaggelis did this and was advised everything regarding the blood vessels was in order.

At this stage the doctor told him he had psychological issues and recommended Vaggelis visit a psychologist. The doctor prescribed him Cialis to help with his feelings.

# At this point Vaggelis felt he had no hope to be treated.

The Cialis tablets caused huge prostate pains and Vaggelis knew it was not psychological problems, so he visited another doctor. This new doctor said he had an infection in his prostate and advised he undertake a blood and sperm examination. When he did the examination, they found chlamydia. The doctor prescribed the pill Vibramycin for one month. Vaggelis started to feel better, and for once he did not have a burning feeling while urinating. However, when he stopped taking Vibramycin, after one week the symptoms returned. He went back to the same doctor and was advised to take two more weeks of Vibramycin. This time the symptoms did not disappear.

He went to this doctor a third time and let him know that his symptoms remained. The doctor did an ultrasound and advised Vaggelis did not have an infection anymore. At this point the doctor recommended treatment with PiezoWaves on the prostate and penis and said everything would be fine and he would recover.

Each cycle of PiezoWaves was six sessions. In total Vaggelis did three cycles, meaning eighteen treatments in total. The doctor also recommended some herbs and supplements, including Epimedium Macun.

Sometimes while on the herbs Vaggelis would notice while reading that white pages were turning blue; he also had a humming sensation in his ears. He was very disappointed the PiezoWaves and herbs did not work after a treatment period of over nine months. The doctor said to wait another six months for results and to be patient.

At this stage Vaggelis felt very bad from a mental perspective and really felt nobody could cure him. He also split up with his girlfriend at this point as she was feeling that his erectile dysfunction was maybe a sign he was not attracted to her anymore.

Vaggelis then stopped visiting doctors for a long time and started doing research on other solutions. He found some mushrooms called Ganoderma which assisted with the symptoms but did not cure the problem.

Vaggelis found Dr Pavlos Georgiadis on the internet in 2020 and visited him after the first lockdowns in May 2020.

## Treatment

The doctor examined Vaggelis very carefully via transrectal examination and an ultrasound of the testicles, bladder, kidneys and abdomen.

The doctor advised Vaggelis he had a big Chronic Prostatitis problem with lots of inflammation shown on the transrectal prostate scan. He also diagnosed a varicocele (an enlargement of the veins within the loose bag of skin that holds the testicles). His uroflow test showed a very weak average urinary flow of 5.5 ml per second with lots of interruptions.

His sperm test results showed that staphylococcus epimedium and E. coli were present at high levels. Vaggelis started two prostate massages per day in June 2020. These massages were painful at first due to his haemorrhoids, and lasted throughout the months of June and July.

After two weeks of prostate massages, Vaggelis stopped waking up to pee at night and his sperm quantity was raised. At the end of July 2020, he had his first intraprostatic injection. After a two-month break to work and save funds, Vaggelis came back to Athens in October 2020; he continued twice-daily prostate massages until November 2020. Vaggelis then took a nine-month break from the program to focus on his work and property rentals.

In September 2021, Vaggelis started twice-daily prostate massages again for three weeks in preparation for his second intraprostatic injection. This second injection was done in October 2021. From October 2021 to December 2021 Vaggelis had one prostate massage per day.

He then stopped the treatment program for six months due to work and personal priorities and started eating in a less healthy manner. During his six months break from the program Vaggelis started eating traditional Crete-style rice with butter, desserts with sweet bread and cheese, lots of local honey and occasional wine and cocktails. (These are exactly the types of food not recommended to be consumed by Chronic Prostatitis sufferers.)

Vaggelis came back to the clinic in Athens in June 2022 for an examination and his prostate had grown 5 ml larger due to his poor diet while off the program.

He started one prostate massage a day and became stricter on the foods he consumed. A third intraprostatic injection is planned for 2023.

Overall Vaggelis currently feels much better than he did. He has better control of urination and has better erections. Psychologically he knows he is on a path to recovery and now feels hope.

This is vastly different to his peak of symptoms.

At one point in 2020, Vaggelis was on a flight from Thessaloniki to Athens and he thought to himself, what if the plane crashes? His answer was he didn't really care, because at that stage everything in his life felt so bad.

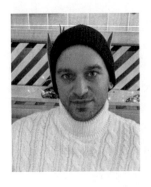

## George's story (thirty-four years old)

### Summary

George's symptoms started when he was twenty-three. At the time he was living in a shared student house that was not that clean. He had a relationship with a fellow student who was rebellious and did not have the best oral hygiene.

The first symptom George experienced was frequent urination with a burning sensation. He visited a doctor who gave him some pills, as the burning urination was really annoying him. George took the pills for three weeks but never really felt 100% better. He visited the doctor again who said George was fine despite him still not feeling great.

George carried on trying not to worry about his symptoms. In 2012, George was on a long bus journey in Turkey that took twelve hours. There was no toilet on the bus and George was in excruciating pain to urinate. He eventually urinated in a plastic bottle at the back of the bus and was surprised to find only a very small amount actually came out of him. His relief was huge, but it seemed strange to him he was in so much pain for such little urine output.

By the middle of 2013, George returned to Greece and joined the Army. By now he was urinating small amounts ten or eleven times a day. George went to see a psychologist in the army given he was urinating so much and was starting to feel stressed. The psychologist had no meaningful feedback to provide.

He went to another doctor in the Army who prescribed some tablets at the military hospital. George took all three boxes over a few weeks but nothing much happened. He possibly urinated a little faster.

In 2015, George moved to Berlin and for three years was not living a healthy lifestyle. He was clubbing quite a lot, drinking excessively and not resting or eating well. His frequent urination made him very anxious and less confident. He felt like he started to develop psychological problems and excess worry.

By the time George was twenty-six or twenty-seven, he was starting to have some sexual dysfunction problems. He visited a psychologist in Germany but was very shy to tell his story.

By 2019, George started to just live with his symptoms and just thought the stress, alcohol and partying in his life was just not good for him. He felt much better when exercising, partying less and eating healthier.

George still had burning during urination and very frequent urination. By now he had also started to experience very sharp pains in his lower abdomen.

## George started to think he had cancer, and was starting to think very dark thoughts due to his painful symptoms.

The symptoms were always on George's mind and it was taking his energy. He did not express his feelings to his parents, friends or girlfriends and kept all the problems in his head.

During 2022 George decided to visit a urologist who did a urine test.

## The doctor said George had Chronic Prostatitis. He advised, 'you just have to live with it, it's a pain in the arse'.

The urologist gave George some antibiotics and said you won't be cured but you will feel some relief. George started to urinate better after the tablets but the effect soon wore off and the symptoms started again.

By the summer of 2022 George could not even sit down peacefully. He felt as if something was inflamed between his legs. Also, sometimes when he pooed, white liquid would come out of his penis. This really worried George.

By November 2022, George was starting to feel a very strong pain in his abdomen and arranged to visit Dr Pavlos Georgiadis in Athens.

## Treatment

The doctor performed a transrectal scan on George on 15 December 2022. The scan showed strong inflammation in George's prostate. George also had a sperm culture test performed, which showed staphylococcus aureus, enterobacter cloacae and ureaplasma urealyticum were present.

George started twice-daily prostate massages in January 2023 and is starting to feel fewer symptoms, and feels as if he is on a path to getting his life back.

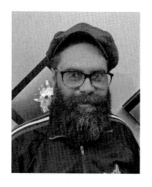

# Thomas's story (thirty-four years old)

## Summary

Five years ago, Thomas was returning from a seaside trip and stopped off the main road to pee. He noticed when he urinated a painful and burning feeling. He thought it would be a temporary feeling, however when he returned home and urinated again, he felt the same pain.

He also noticed that night when he went to bed that he had a temperature. With the temperature and urinary burning sensation Thomas decided to visit a hospital late at night. He wanted immediate treatment as he was worried about these symptoms.

He had a urine test done and after two hours the doctor diagnosed Prostatitis. He was given some antibiotics to take. After ten days of antibiotics, he was feeling fine and didn't seek any further treatment.

Three years later Thomas had surgery on his knee. While in hospital he had to urinate in a plastic bottle as he was confined to a wheelchair after the knee operation. Four to five days after the surgery on his knee Thomas noticed while at home that the burning feeling during urination started again.

He started the process of getting checked over again and went to his local doctor. The doctor requested he do a scan on his abdomen and organs. Everything was fine and perfectly normal according to the scans the doctor advised.

He then went to see a local urologist and his adventure officially started. The urologist gave Thomas some coloured plastic pieces to urinate on to test him for the presence of bacteria. The doctor said that if the colours changed on the test it indicated bacteria were present.

Following the test, the doctor said Thomas had bacteria and prescribed him some more antibiotics. After two weeks of these antibiotics some of Thomas's symptoms went away but they did not go completely.

Following these antibiotics, Thomas started to notice a pain in his left testicle for the first time. After a week of this testicle pain Thomas mentioned this to his doctor. His doctor alarmingly said: 'Maybe your testicles are banging together during sex, causing this pain.'

After two more weeks Thomas noticed red spots in his sperm he had never seen before when he ejaculated. He was very worried about this and relayed this to his doctor when he called him on his mobile phone one Sunday. The situation was becoming more stressful for Thomas, and he was starting to worry about what the problem was more and more.

The doctor prescribed yet more antibiotics, but given this doctor did not seem to be giving the right answers he tried another doctor. He explained the situation to his new doctor, who explained Thomas needed to do a sperm and urine test. He did the sperm test and the result that came back was he had an E. coli infection.

The doctor gave Thomas an additional pill, Arrenprost, to take after a meal daily, together with some daily antibiotics. The doctor said that 'with this new pill, and the antibiotics we will exterminate the bacteria'.

Thomas kept taking these antibiotics for five months, but he was still having symptoms, stress and pain.

During the Easter period of 2021, Thomas contracted COVID and noticed his sperm around this time was a strange heavy yellowy–green colour. The doctor advised this was because of the recent COVID infection.

Thomas also visited another urologist around this time, who scanned his prostate. The urologist said Thomas's prostate was inflamed but was generally a good size. The prostate inflammation was nothing to worry about, he was advised.

Thomas had started visiting the internet by now to do his own research and found Dr Pavlos Georgiadis. He was quickly convinced this was the most serious doctor and called to arrange an appointment in September 2022. To Thomas's surprise Pavlos answered the phone late at night when Thomas called the clinic.

The doctor suggested he visit with a full bladder so he could perform a uroflow test. Pavlos also performed a prostate transrectal scan and prostate massage, followed by a sperm test at a local microbiological laboratory.

The results showed Thomas had E. coli and enterococcus bacteria in his prostate. His prostate scan showed severe red inflammation. The doctor advised Thomas he had likely had Prostatitis for over ten years but was asymptomatic for much of this.

## Treatment

Thomas has started daily prostate massages and is starting to improve already. His urinary burning is reducing and testicle pain is diminishing.

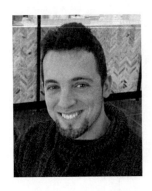

## Hamit's story (thirty-one years old)

### Summary

At twenty-eight years old, Hamit started to feel sick and in a low mood. He was starting to feel very tired at work.

He did not pay much attention to it as these feelings were only temporary. Hamit could do his work fitting aluminum windows and go to the gym perfectly fine. However, one month he had to stop going to the gym as he felt so tired and down. This tiredness continued for two years.

The next symptom he encountered was an irritation during ejaculation. At this time his twenty-four-year-old girlfriend had some problems, including fungi and sinus problems. She persuaded Hamit to visit a urologist.

The urologist did not impose any tests on him. The doctor advised Hamit he was very young and said maybe the pain was from his work and standing up a lot.

Hamit insisted on being examined. The doctor did a simple ultrasound and told him that his prostate was fine. The doctor said to relieve Hamit's stress he should also do a urine test, which showed all was fine.

He left the urologist feeling assured, but it didn't last long. After a few months ejaculation became even more painful for a period of two minutes afterwards. He also started to feel even more tired. At night he could not fall asleep easily and was not sleeping well. He constantly woke up in the morning tired.

At this stage Hamit looked in the bathroom mirror each morning; he noticed a few grey hairs on his head and said to himself at thirty-one, 'I got old'.

He then started to notice a drop in the intensity of his urination, however he was unable to distinguish all these symptoms as a problem on his own.

He decided to put it all out of his mind and for a year did not think about it. This was until he had another symptom that disturbed him. The next symptom was erections of a very short duration. By now he was also starting to urinate frequently at night.

By the summer of 2022, Hamit arranged to see a different urologist and advised him about his erectile dysfunction. This urologist told Hamit to do a sperm culture test but did not submit him to anyone to do the test. He undertook one though his own initiative and it came back positive for staphylococcus haemolyticus.

The doctor prescribed Hamit to take a week's course of Ciproxin antibiotics. Taking the antibiotics took all Hamit's symptoms away except the regular urination. The doctor advised he was fine and now cured. Hamit felt relieved and happy at this point.

After taking these antibiotics Hamit's tendons in his arm started to hurt and his stomach also generated some pain. Nevertheless, for two months he felt well, little by little. However, soon the symptoms started to reappear one by one.

By now the symptoms were becoming more and more intense to the point of affecting his daily life at work. After two to three hours of standing, Hamit had severe pain in the groin and a feeling of weight in his testicles.

Hamit called the doctor again, who told him the whole problem was psychological and suggested giving him pills to sleep and for better psychology.

Hamit just could not accept medication for his psychology. He started to feel very frustrated and undertook his own research on the internet. He found many doctors and urologists on the internet but most of them only prescribed drugs in their protocol. The only options to get better according to this research were pills or surgery.

In September 2022, Hamit then found Dr Pavlos Georgiadis website and read further about his protocol.

## Treatment

Hamit visited the doctor initially on 20 September 2022. On arrival at the doctor's clinic, he immediately performed some thorough examinations, including:

- transrectal scan of prostate
- testicle scan
- abdomen, kidney and bladder scan
- urine uroflow test
- prostate massage followed by visiting a special laboratory for a sperm culture test.

These examinations showed that Hamit had Chronic Prostatitis caused by staphylococcus haemolyticus, which the doctor diagnosed had probably been in his prostate for six to ten years.

His prostate scan showed significant inflammation and infection. His urinary flow was very low at a maximum rate of 14.1 ml per second.

Hamit felt very safe being diagnosed, and after his first prostate massage started to feel better, even though he passed out. The first prostate massage was very tough and he sweated a lot.

Since November 2022, Hamit has been having twice-daily prostate massages and once-daily PiezoWave prostate treatment. He has had one intraprostatic injection which took place on 20 December 2022.

While Hamit still has some way to go on his treatment program he is already feeling in excellent condition. He feels stronger, happier, and sex is better again. He is sleeping better, feels less anxious and now does not get tired like he used to.

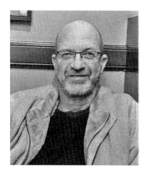

## Paul's story (fifty-nine years old)

### Summary

Paul's symptoms started with pain after ejaculating and an uncomfortable feeling in his testicles at forty-nine years old during 2013. Paul also remembers having premature ejaculation from a much earlier age of around twenty-three. After two years he went to see a urologist because of these symptoms.

The urologist unexpectedly sent Paul to have his prostate measured. The results were that he had an enlarged prostate. The doctor said there was medicine for this but it would not cure it. The doctor also advised Paul he did not need to take the medicine, so Paul didn't.

The doctor also asked Paul about his urination and Paul advised him he urinates twice at night and every two hours during the day.

Paul continued to have pain from ejaculation and he was also starting to notice he didn't want to get an erection very often.

In 2015 Paul's girlfriend wasn't very happy about Paul's erectile issues as they were trying for a baby. Paul had started to notice his sperm was weak and his partner at this time unfortunately had a miscarriage. The stress on the relationship caused the couple to split, and by 2018 when he had a new girlfriend Paul was ejaculating very quickly during sexual encounters. Due to the pain Paul did not want to have sex frequently.

Paul remembers going to a hotel with his girlfriend and feeling that he needed to meticulously plan any sexual situation. His girlfriend mentioned there was a pill and cream he could take to delay ejaculation but Paul decided not to regularly use this. Generally, after ejaculation Paul felt extremely weak the next day.

By August 2018, Paul was urinating very frequently. Once while visiting the US, he had to carefully plan his daily bathroom trips to friendly restaurants with bathrooms. Although he was urinating frequently between August 2018 and August 2019, Paul did not consider his urination a problem.

By May 2020, when Paul took on a new job as a computer engineer, it was a stressful time and his urination became worse.

## Paul started to urinate every fifty minutes.

This frequent urination carried on and also became accompanied with a very strong burning sensation that was causing Paul real suffering. Paul went to a doctor who recommended Xatral, an alpha blocker to relax the urination. Paul did not take the tablets as the doctor said a side effect would be to not have sperm. Paul also did not want to put chemicals in his body.

In 2020, Paul started Chinese therapy with acupuncture and herbs, which helped reduce the burning from intense to mediocre. Paul continued with a combination of Chinese and Korean medicine between May 2020 and November 2020, and it helped reduce the burning sensation. Paul however still did not feel 100% healthy.

## By 2021, Paul was experiencing an extremely strong burning pain after ejaculation.

### Treatment

Paul was recommended to Dr Pavlos Georgiadis by a friend and Paul did further research on the internet.

In November 2022, Paul visited Dr Georgiadis who discovered Paul had a significantly enlarged and inflamed prostate and the presence of two types of staphylococcus bacteria in his prostate.

As I write this, Paul has had several weeks of treatment and is feeling that he is happier and in the right place for treatment. While

Paul still has a burning sensation while urinating, he is able to urinate over a period of a minute when it previously took seven or eight minutes.

Daily prostate massages are easier to bear, his urination is improving and Paul feels he is on the road to getting his life back.

## John's Story (forty years old)

### Summary

John first noticed symptoms at twenty-six years old, which was a difficulty in urinating. At this time John was a strong guy who worked out at the gym three times a week, he regularly put on gym weightlifters' pants to protect his testicles during heavy weightlifting sessions. (On reflection John believes his original infection was caused by using these dirty weightlifters' pants as he was fully protected during any sexual encounters around this time.)

One year later he noticed problems getting an erection as well as a noticeably decreased libido. He went to see a doctor in 2010 who said John had weak blood flow in his penis but did not give a reason for it.

Due to his erection difficulties and reduced libido, John's psychology was getting worse and worse. It affected his everyday behaviour and he became depressed. These heavy psychological symptoms also caused him stomach pains and further stress.

John had become very depressed and his doctor prescribed him Ladose antidepressant pills which made his libido and sexual dysfunction even worse. Nevertheless, John continued to take the Ladose tablets between 2014 and 2018.

In 2018, John went to see another doctor who said John had Chronic Pelvic Pain syndrome as by now he was experiencing severe pain in his pelvis and back. John wasn't prescribed anything by this doctor so he went to the doctor in his local town, who thought he may have an infection and prescribed some antibiotics. These antibiotics did not really help or reduce symptoms.

In 2022, John visited one more doctor and took antibiotics for two more months. This doctor also tried to persuade John to do piezo shockwave treatment on his penis which he did not want to do.

## Treatment

In January 2022, John came to visit Dr Pavlos Georgiadis as his last hope to get better. He is undertaking daily prostate massages and is already starting to see reduced symptoms and is feeling healthier.

## Spiros's story (fifty-five years old)

### Summary

At the end of 2001 when he was thirty-three years old Spiros got an infection after a sexual encounter. He had an itching sensation when urinating and a general pain around the penis. He was surprised with these symptoms and didn't know what it was.

He left things several weeks as he thought it was only minor and that it would go away.

After a few weeks Spiros went to see a doctor. The doctor did examinations in the form of a urine culture and semen culture test. The results showed E. coli was present in his urine.

Spiros was prescribed Ciprofloxacin antibiotics. He took the antibiotics for two to three weeks but did not experience any relief from the symptoms. Spiros believes, looking back and after doing some research, that his eating yoghurt straight after the tablets may have made them ineffective.

He went back to the doctor who prescribed Norocin tablets this time. These tablets worked very well over a period of three weeks.

After three weeks when he stopped the tablets the symptoms came back, but this time the symptoms were even stronger. He was now experiencing pain in his thighs, felt very tired, had pain in his lower abdomen and overall body aches. The symptoms were similar to fibromyalgia he noted during our discussion.

His doctor said he should keep on taking Norocin, which Spiros reluctantly continued for two to three months. The tablets did not really help with his symptoms.

He started to accept the symptoms and started exploring other doctors.

The next doctor he visited in the summer of 2002 was a rheumatologist who diagnosed fibromyalgia and prescribed some minerals to relax his muscles, including magnesium, and some light antidepressants.

At this stage aside from his symptoms and tiredness, Spiros was starting to feel very worried.

He started these new medicines and noticed improvements after a month, with less pain in the body and the leg, and his foot pain went away. He was still getting pain when urinating.

The problem with the antidepressants was they constantly made him want to sleep. One night he fell asleep at 9 pm before a 10 pm work call. When he awoke for the phone call his jaw was too relaxed to even talk.

By 2003 Spiros decided to stop taking all tablets and little by little his symptoms seemed to improve. For the period between 2003 and 2008 Spiros had almost no symptoms except occasional minor penis pain. All the way up to 2020 Spiros was living normally, with minor symptoms that didn't affect his life. Spiros would have mild penis discomfort once a month but did not want to go back on to antibiotics or other tablets.

In the summer of 2020 Spiros had unprotected sex. The next day he had pain on urination, pain in the back and overall was not feeling well. All the original symptoms from 2001 returned.

At this stage he did not know what to do. He went to a doctor again. The doctor prescribed Norocin. Spiros took the Norocin for four weeks. The symptoms reduced but did not disappear. After the four weeks of Norocin antibiotics Spiros stopped them, but the symptoms continued for another year. He had constant pain in his back, pain in his legs and overall lethargy.

In 2020, Spiros found Dr Pavlos Georgiadis on the internet but was unable to visit him as he was living in Portugal and COVID-19 was restricting travel.

## Treatment

Finally, in June 2021 Spiros had his first meeting with the doctor and was thoroughly examined.

The sperm culture test on Spiros showed that the staphylococcus bacteria was present in his prostate. From June 2021, Spiros did three weeks of twice-daily prostate massages followed by an intraprostatic injection. Due to work commitments and living abroad, Spiros then took a two-month break before repeating the same three weeks of prostate massages followed by an intraprostatic injection.

Spiros has to date undertaken four sets of three weeks of prostate massages followed by an intraprostatic injection during the course of 2021 and 2022.

He has already noticed a considerable improvement in the way he feels and says, 'I now feel quite normal'. He still gets some minor perennial pain and minor itching during urination, but overall feels way better.

Spiros is looking forward to finishing his treatment in the mid-term and is determined to get his life back.

# William's story (twenty-one years old)

## Summary

At nineteen William felt a burning sensation when urinating and he needed to urinate very frequently. He was going to pee around eight times a day.

This carried on for two weeks, during which time William tried to forget about it. He also felt embarrassed to talk to his parents about this.

Eventually he opened up to his parents, who said let's go to see a urologist. William went to a urologist the family knew who did a lower abdomen ultrasound. The doctor asked William where he was experiencing the pain and his reply was at the base of the penis. The doctor told him not to worry, we will do a urine sample at a laboratory.

The urologist gave William a paper to get a government-subsidised urine test and wrote on the paper the reason for the test was suspected Chronic Prostatitis. The urologist did not mention this to William, he just noted it on the urination sample advice note.

When William questioned the laboratory about this on arrival, they said don't worry we need a reason listed to undertake a urination test. When the urine test results came back, they showed positive for klebsiella pneumoniae.

Given the test was taken at a government laboratory, William then called the doctor and advised the result, which the doctor could now see on his screen. The doctor prescribed Ciproxin antibiotics for three weeks. William started to take the antibiotics and after three weeks he was feeling much better and didn't have symptoms. He felt back to normal.

After the three weeks on antibiotics and twenty days off them, William did a second urine test. The test showed positive for no microbiological bacteria.

Two months after this William felt that he was relapsing. First came the urge to urinate more, the burning sensation was worse, and when William sat in a specific way on a hard chair or gym bicycle there was a pain radiating in the base of his penis.

At this point William went to see a second urologist who recommended a urine test and sperm test. The results showed he had staphylococcus aureus and chlamydia.

William started taking antibiotics again but this time they were Augmentin and Rulide. After twenty-eight days of antibiotics, William waited another twenty days off the antibiotics before visiting the urologist again. He did another urine and sperm test which this time showed no chlamydia but that staphylococcus aureus was still present.

These tests were done at the Mycolab laboratory. Mycolab advised William, ideally, they needed three clean results to fully confirm chlamydia is out of his system. They also advised staphylococcus aureus needs antibiotics, despite many doctors and urologists saying it is a natural microbe in the body.

By now William's urge to urinate and pain while sitting were still annoying, so he went to see a third urologist. This urologist said you are very young to have taken so many antibiotics. We don't want your body to become resistant to these tablets that may be needed later in your life.

## The urologist then said, 'It's all in your mind, and I recommended you forget about it and relax.'

The urologist also advised William to not sit in a chair for too long and to not continue using an exercise bicycle at the gym.

Another month passed and the symptoms were still annoying him. William called Mycolab and advised about the lack of progress; they advised he needed to find a urologist who understands the problem and who prescribes the right antibiotics.

William then visited his fourth urologist, who said they don't prescribe antibiotics for this. William pushed for a solution as he was becoming more anxious and stressed, and he was given Augmentin for three weeks.

After three weeks of tablets the symptoms were exactly the same – the tablets did not make a difference. William started to think, *I'm too young for this and should not be getting this sitting and back pain.*

Two additional months passed and William maintained a good diet, drank lots of water and exercised regularly. He had started to live with the symptoms and normalise them in his mind.

Now the urge to urinate became worse and the pain when sitting was even stronger. William also started to notice a pain when ejaculating, and thought to himself *I really now need to make an effort to deal with this.*

He wanted to find a doctor that did more than just hand out antibiotics and found Dr. Pavlos Georgiadis online.

## Treatment

William first visited Dr Georgiadis in April 2022 for analytical examinations, including a transrectal scan, ultrasound, uroflow urine test and sperm culture test following a prostate massage.

The doctor was able to show William on a screen that his prostate was inflamed and infected. He also explained he had a minor urinary obstruction. The sperm test results came back positive for staphylococcus aureus and klebsiella pneumoniae.

William started treatment in April 2022, comprising one prostate massage a day along with Augmentin and Norocin antibiotics.

After two weeks of treatment William was feeling much better. He then took an Easter break and did further prostate massages in May 2022. He was now on a very healthy diet and his symptoms were getting far better. There was no sitting pain problem and not so much urination needed.

After a summer vacation, William restarted treatment in early September 2022 for two-and-a-half weeks. He also had a second sperm culture test performed. The sperm test showed the staphylococcus aureus was present at lower levels and the klebsiella pneumoniae had been eradicated.

His studies from October to December took William overseas and he returned again to prostate massages, this time twice-daily from January 2023.

William's prostate is already 3 ml smaller and he is feeling at his top level again. He does not have constant symptoms and only very occasionally gets burning during urination. He is feeling happy and ambitious again and is looking forward to finishing the program and getting his life back.

Looking back, William is convinced that swimming in a dirty public swimming pool when he was eighteen years old was the start of his infection and problems.

## Vassilis's story (thirty years old)

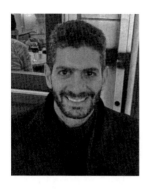

### Summary

Vassilis started to suffer from terrible headaches, which he described as a 'headache crisis' during September and October 2016. He went for several examinations, including at a neurologist, pathologist and ear, nose and throat specialist. These examinations included undertaking an MRI scan on his brain.

All of these specialists said Vassilis had no problem and was perfectly fine. The headache symptoms suddenly disappeared in March 2017. Vassilis put these headaches down to tough times while he was studying and carried on his life for a year-and-a-half with no problems.

In December 2018, Vassilis started to notice some erection problems that lasted for four days. He visited a urologist and underwent a doppler examination – the urologist said there were no problems with Vassilis's urogenital system.

Life was then normal for six months and he thought these erectile issues were just due to stress and tiredness.

In January 2019, Vassilis went overseas to study and was living a normal life until one day he vividly recalls. It was 1 June 2019 and Vassilis woke up with pain from his ankles, all over his back bones right up to his neck. His headaches were much more intense than before, which caused Vassilis to get really upset as he just did not know what the problem was.

Vassilis could not stand. He could not walk. All he wanted to do was lay in bed and stay the whole day as the pain was so intense.

Vassilis explained to me: 'I really thought something bad was going on.'

This extreme pain carried on for twenty days. During this time Vassilis started to research disabled persons' jobs for the future as he was convinced it would be a long-term disability.

While he stayed at home unable to walk, Vassilis realised the pain was coming from between his legs. He did more research on the internet and was convinced it was something to do with his urological system.

He then visited a urologist in Belgium who said he had no problem. This was followed up with a meeting with urologists in the Netherlands and Germany, who both said there was no issue.

In June 2019, Vassilis came back to Greece and started visiting more urologists; he recalls visiting six or seven urologists in total, which included some very famous professors.

None of these urologists did a very detailed examination of Vassilis and all of them said he had psychological problems and should visit a psychologist. The final urologist sent Vassilis for an examination at a diagnostic centre which did a urine test that showed no infection or problems. Vassilis was told by this last urologist:

You need to redefine your nature as a man,
because something is wrong with you.

In September 2019, Vassilis visited a psychologist for the first time. His sessions over video call were designed to help him get used to everyday life with his pain. The psychologist said, 'I cannot do anything for your pain, but I can help you to find ways to make the pain part of your everyday life … this is your life from now on, so you need to find ways to get used to it.'

Vassilis was still in so much pain he could not live a normal life of seeing friends, going to restaurants and the things normal people do.

## Treatment

By the end of December 2019, Vassilis reached out to Dr Pavlos Georgiadis as his last hope. He set an appointment for 7 January 2020 with the doctor, who did a careful examination of Vassilis, including a transrectal scan, abdomen scan and laboratory sperm test.

His transrectal prostate scan showed a very inflamed prostate (with lots of red spots) that was 15 ml in size. The doctor however said it was important to find out if bacteria was causing this inflammation.

On 20 January 2020 (Vassilis's birthday), Vassilis vividly recalls getting his sperm test results which showed staphylococcus aureus bacteria was present.

## Vassilis started celebrating with delight when he found out he had bacteria present in his prostate.

This confirmed to Vassilis that he was not crazy and did not have psychological issues after all. He knew all along there was something wrong with him and was relieved to now have an accurate diagnosis.

After 20 January 2020, Vassilis's psychology became better every day. Vassilis started the Chronic Prostatitis rejuvenation program on 13 February 2020 and after his third prostate massage 80% of his symptoms had disappeared. He was starting to get back to a normal life.

During 2020 and 2021 Vassilis had sixteen injections in his prostate to kill a total of eight bacterial microbes that were discovered. He has had no microbiological bacteria in his prostate since May 2022 and has been symptom free since July 2020.

Vassilis's prostate has reduced to 10 ml in size, but more importantly he has gotten his life back.

## Victor's story (thirty-three years old)

### Summary

In 2017, Victor went to get his sperm count checked as he had been trying for a baby with his wife. The sperm check showed Victor only had 20% moveable penetrating sperm, which was a very low count. He had an ultrasonic prostate scan done and was advised his prostate was inflamed in many places.

This infertility clinic recommended a blood examination and penile shaft smear test. The smear test discovered bacteria proteus was present. Victor was prescribed some antibiotics and the bacteria subsided.

After these antibiotics Victor's sperm count measured 29% and his prostate was less inflamed. He was advised by the fertility clinic to drink more herbal teas to continue reducing the prostate inflammation.

One year after this in 2018, Victor's first real symptoms started. He had inflamed urinary channels and burning when peeing. Victor went to a urologist this time and was prescribed antibiotics, from which he felt some quick relief.

However, after this Victor was noticing whenever he was drinking beers with friends in the months that followed, he woke up in the morning with the feeling of knives in his lower stomach and anus. The symptoms got worse through 2018 and Victor was having to urinate ten to fifteen times a day. Victor went to another clinic and was given some more antibiotics to take and advised he would soon be better.

By this time Victor's left leg was tingling a lot so he went to a nerve doctor who explained it could be because of stress. He was prescribed some Apaurin to reduce stress. Victor did not take these as he did not want to take antidepressant-type pills.

Victor's peeing problems continued and he had a burning while urinating. Several other doctors prescribed antibiotics which calmed down the burning a little bit but did not stop the urination frequency.

In early 2019, Victor had started road cycling regularly but he had such terrible pain in the anus and penis when cycling he had to stop the hobby. He was also working out at a gym frequently but had to stop this due to feeling lethargic.

In 2020, Victor went back to the original clinic. He did another prostate scan; this time his prostate was even more inflamed and red on the image he was shown. He also did a sperm analysis which showed E. coli bacteria was present and his moveable sperm count was down to 5%. Victor was given antibiotics for six months to eradicate the E. coli, however after three weeks further tests showed the E. coli were resistant to the antibiotics.

Victor's next doctor prescribed intravenous antibiotics twice a day, which resulted in a cleaner 26% sperm count. Finally, Victor was happy having a better sperm count and less symptoms.

Victor started to eat normally and live normally but within a month his symptoms returned. Victor by now had strong pelvic pain, leg tingling, peeing problems, dry mouth, red eyes, rash on arms, pain in lower back and general melancholy.

Victor felt like he was not getting anywhere with urologists so in 2021 he decided to visit different specialists. Victor visited specialists for a colonoscopy, gastroscopy and a scan of the abdomen. These checks showed Victor had a spasm in his bowel and Chronic Prostatitis.

After this Victor visited seven different doctors who all said they could not cure Chronic Prostatitis but all were willing to offer antibiotics.

Victor was struggling for solutions by now and started to drink natural teas with probiotics which his friend who was a doctor recommended. Victor was also on a healthy diet and drank no alcohol. After three months Victor felt some relief and everything subsided except penile burning up to Christmas 2022.

During Christmas in 2022 with family and friends Victor drank some alcohol and ate all the festive food. His symptoms came back, with extreme pain in the pelvic area.

At this point Victor did not know what to do and found Dr Pavlos Georgiadis on the internet.

## Treatment

In March 2023, Victor came to visit Dr Pavlos Georgiadis as his last hope. His prostate scan showed extreme prostate inflammation and the presence of pseudomonas aeruginosa, morganella morganii and chlamydia bacteria. Victor commenced his first few prostate massages and is already finding the extreme pain is diminishing.

Victor is planning to come back to Greece for a more intensive treatment program now he knows there is a solution to getting his life back.

# George's story (thirty-seven years old)

## Summary

In September 2018, George came down with a really bad fever, had absolutely no energy and noticed blood in his urine. He visited his doctor for what would be the first of over fifteen times in total over the coming three years. During his first doctor's visit George was prescribed Ciprofloxacin antibiotics which made his symptoms subside, and after ten days' rest, he was feeling better.

However, seven months later a really bad fever came back again, this time accompanied by back pain and left testicle pain. George was told to rest and was prescribed Ciprofloxacin again.

Two months later, George had a fever again and was back at the doctor. These episodes of bad fever, intermittent blood in urine and terrible lethargy would come on every three to six months.

George's prostate was also starting to feel tight, and he had pain all down his left leg from his left testicle. He also found his sharpness of mind and creativity disappeared and it was difficult for him to focus.

All of these symptoms made things psychologically difficult for George, and he felt very down. He stopped working on his new business venture and had to stop his outside sporting interests such as kickboxing and football. George would feel really tired even after doing a small amount of computer administration work.

George felt like he had only 20% of his normal mind power.

In July 2021, while on vacation George visited a different doctor in his home country of Greece who prescribed two months of antibiotics. George took these antibiotics and started a healthier diet and felt great for the next year and a half. Then once again the fever came back to hit him hard in December 2022. George broke down crying and was starting to get really scared about what was the matter with him.

## Psychologically he was not in a great place.

George would have to completely stop work for two or three weeks at a time and his family were starting to notice a difference in him. They could tell he was really down and even a pleasant experience like a vacation was often interrupted with doctors' visits. Family drives were also a problem given the pain in George's back and legs.

By the end of 2022 George had had enough and decided to visit Dr Pavlos Georgiadis, who he had seen online.

### Treatment

George's fist examination from Dr Pavlos Georgiadis showed a heavily swollen prostate through a transrectal scan. His sperm test showed the presence of chlamydia and E. coli.

George has started twice-daily prostate massages and has had one antibiotic injection in his prostate. His inflammation has already significantly reduced, he is looking healthier and feeling more energetic.

George is confident he will get his life back and make his small company he put on hold a success.

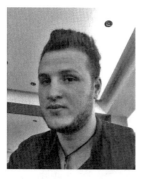

# Eralds's story (thirty-one years old)

## Summary

In 2018, Erald started to notice pain in his testicles, especially when he walked. He had also been getting burning while urinating before this but ignored it as he thought it was normal. But over the next few months, the pain in his testicles became stronger and spread to his legs and lower back.

Erald went to a doctor who did an external ultrasound check and said everything was okay.

The pain became even stronger so Erald went to another doctor. This doctor said he had a mild infection in his prostate but would be fine.

The doctor gave Erald three weeks of antibiotics and said all the symptoms would go away. Erald took the antibiotics and felt a little bit of an improvement but still had underlying pain.

He went back to the same doctor who changed his antibiotic type and gave him another three weeks' worth to take. After taking this second batch of antibiotics the situation was still the same.

By now Erald was getting pain in the urethra area inside his body, he had pain in his testicles even more and pain in his legs. His testicles were even painful when he touched them.

Erald changed doctors again and this new one did a sperm test, which showed bacteria was present and that his spermogram number was low. This doctor said Erald had a problem and wanted to do surgery as he said Erald had a varicocele (an enlargement of the veins within the loose bag of skin that holds the testicles).

This doctor gave Erald some Bactrimel antibiotics to take for one month. After taking these antibiotics Erald felt relaxed and fine for two to three months.

Soon however the symptoms came back even worse, with a strong burning pain after ejaculation and even stronger leg, back and testicle pain.

## Day by day the pain was getting even worse.

Erald went to another doctor as he did not want any surgery. This next doctor said Erald had psychological problems and also gave him Buscopan tablets for his now worsening stomach problems.

By this stage Erald was feeling very nervous and becoming more stressed regarding what his problem really was. Erald was now urinating much more frequently, around ten times during the day and five times at night.

Erald went to another doctor who diagnosed that Erald had Chronic Prostatitis but said he would have to live with it. This doctor said to Erald he would have to get used to this as it is not curable. This doctor recommended three months of antibiotics, which Erald took. When he stopped taking these antibiotics his body literally shook from pain.

## Erald had to stop his job as he could not work, was always tired and could not concentrate properly.

In January 2020, Erald was visiting family in Greece and he went to visit a private doctor while there. This doctor said to Erald he will have problems having children if he does not have them now.

While visiting Greece, Erald also decided to visit Dr Pavlos Georgiadis for a second opinion. Dr Pavlos performed a thorough examination of Erald, which showed an extremely inflamed prostate. His urine flow was also restricted, with a maximum flow of only 12 to 13 ml per second when it should be nearer 30 ml per second.

Erald also had three bacteria present in his prostate and was advised he had probably had them for over ten years. Given this took Erald back to when he was sixteen or seventeen years old, before he had sex, Erald could only deduct he had contracted the bacteria from his frequent swimming in a public swimming pool where he grew up in Albania.

## Treatment

Erald started his therapy in January 2020, and within two to three weeks he noticed a big improvement in the way he felt, with the pain significantly reducing due to the prostate massages.

As of writing Erald has received twenty-two prostate injections to break down the terrible inflammation and high levels of long-standing bacteria he had. Erald feels like he is getting his life back and can now function normally. He is looking forward to finishing his treatment and moving forward with his life.

# 7

# PATIENT TREATMENT OPTIONS FOR CHRONIC PROSTATITIS

You will have figured out by now that Chronic Prostatitis is a devastating disease that ruins your quality of life. The key question as a sufferer is, what can you do about it?

I have summarised as best I can below what I would suggest based on the journey that I went through, and cognisant that sufferers are in locations spread right across the world and with differing abilities to get treated from a time and financial perspective.

## Get diagnosed early

Once you have read the range of case studies here to understand what type of symptoms Chronic Prostatitis creates, it is important to get diagnosed early.

The blood and urine tests that I undertook as part of discovering the disease were useless. It is critical you have your sperm analysed by a very professional microbiological laboratory after a specialised massage from a competent and knowledgeable urologist. These competent and knowledgable urologists are hard to find, which is why I ended up being treated in Greece.

I also recommend being very careful with the many western doctors who just hand out antibiotics. As you will have read in the case studies and in my story, tablet antibiotics do not fully penetrate the prostate, where the infection is. Usually stopping antibiotics causes repetition of symptoms, which often come back even stronger.

## Start a healthy diet *immediately*

As you will have read in the case studies, the sufferers who started living a healthier lifestyle were often able to reduce their symptoms. The most substantial thing you can do without treatment to mini-mise symptoms is adopting a careful diet and lifestyle. Avoid sugars, spicy foods, alcohol and in general anything that would increase inflammation. A healthy lifestyle will definitely help with keeping inflammation lower, but the inflammation as well as the microbes will still be there. It is recommended to start an improved diet as soon as you can if you think you have Chronic Prostatitis or have been diagnosed with it.

## Explore newly developing self-massaging technology

Obviously not everyone can make it to Greece for in-person treatment. New technologies such as the prostate probe from www.medoron.com can help patients to self-administer treatment to generate a healthier prostate. This started as a collaboration between senior medical hardware academics from the UK, the clinic in Greece and an international team of Machine Learning postgraduate engineers from UCL and MIT, all with lived experience with Chronic Prostatitis. Their sole mission is to convert Chronic Prostatitis to a globally curable condition, affordably, by enabling protocols based on data-driven objectivity for all men worldwide.

This technology will not fully cure Chronic Prostatitis initially, but it will help soften the prostate and flush out the harmful bacteria causing the inflammation, fibrotic tissue and nerve strangulation.

## Invest in a full treatment program from the Georgiadis Prostate Treatment Protocol

The only global treatment program I am aware of to fully treat Chronic Prostatitis is the Georgiadis protocol that I went through.

As you will have read this treatment for Chronic Prostatitis is difficult, lengthy and can test people's limits, especially considering antibiotics and frequent treatment are involved. In addition, people require the time, money and commitment to visit Athens for sometimes months at a time. This is the fastest way to regain a healthy prostate but also requires the biggest commitment from the patient.

## Investigate what kind of examinations your doctor is using

After talking to many other Chronic Prostatitis sufferers, one other point I would add is for Chronic Prostatitis sufferers to carefully investigate what kind of examinations their doctor is using. Good doctors focus on objectivity, and can prove their results with objective evidence. The other kind of doctors use questionnaires, or stay behind 'what the statistics say', and give patients a diagnosis with very superficial proof, if any.

Only a high-quality transrectal ultrasound with elastography can show an objective snapshot of the prostate at a given time. Radiologists without urological knowledge tend to only check for size and cancer, and ignore Chronic Prostatitis. Urologists without radiological training either don't use transrectal ultrasound or might misuse it.

Microbiological sperm examination needs to happen only after appropriate patient conditioning (prostate massage) and take place at a well-qualified microbiological test clinic.